CLEARING UP SKIN CARE:
A NO-NONSENSE GUIDE TO FINDING A ROUTINE THAT WORKS

Jennifer J. Janiga, MD, FAAD

Janiga MDs
Plastic Surgery and Cosmetic Center
500 Damonte Ranch Pkwy #703
Reno, Nevada 89521

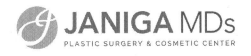

PLASTIC SURGERY & COSMETIC CENTER

ISBN: 9781793495495

Compiled and Formatted by:

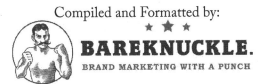

★ ★ ★
BAREKNUCKLE.
BRAND MARKETING WITH A PUNCH

Printed in the United States of America

About the Author

Board-certified dermatologist Dr. Janiga specializes in cosmetic dermatology. Her extensive training and years of experience in medical dermatology, lasers, and cosmetic procedures allow her to treat her patients with the comprehensive attention they deserve.

Patients often describe Dr. Janiga as hardworking, as she won't give up on a problem until a solution is found for the patient. She has a refreshingly simple approach to dermatology: listening attentively to what patients have to say and working with them to plan the right course of action on an individual basis. Honest talk, humility, and a fresh perspective paired with years of experience and education all contribute to the effectiveness of her straightforward care.

Dr. Janiga lives with Dr. Timothy Janiga and her two children in Reno, Nevada (their dream location). In her free time, Dr. Janiga enjoys working out, hiking, reading, and spending time with her family.

Dedication

To my patients: Over the last 20 years, you have taught me humility through your unique and often complex dermatology issues; you have taught me how to discuss your needs in a way that works for you. Most of all you have shown me how powerful family, dedication and community can be. You have made it possible to not only write this book, but to enjoy living by these principles each day.

TABLE OF CONTENTS

DR. JENNIFER JANIGA

INTRODUCTION

The idea for this book originally came about early in my career as a dermatologist when my sister and her friend got to talking about the expenses of skin care. Her friend Claire, a teacher, had recently gone to a day spa in California where she purchased a six-step skin care line in a box. This package of skin care products, which is highly recognized on the market, costs around $550 and lasts about 2 months. Claire liked the products, thought some of them worked, but didn't know which of the six products in the system was the one doing the work. She also felt that the expense was too much for her and her family to be able to continue past the first investment. My sister told her I was a dermatologist and got us together. We had a consultation and reviewed what she liked and didn't like about the products as well as what she was trying to achieve. I suggested a substitute cleanser, dropping one of the products in the line that wasn't specific for her skin problems. I then gave her recommendations on items like antioxidants and a lightening cream that were more specific for her skin. Claire got a skin care system tailored to her needs without compromising quality or effectiveness, and she even removed one product from her routine completely. I checked in on her a few months later and she was happy as could be using a skin care regimen that worked, that was tailored to her and that she could afford to use long term. Now, almost 10 years later, Claire still uses her products, looks great and feels good about how she is spending her money.

My interaction with Claire was a rewarding and educational experience for both of us. I was able to provide this person an effective, custom skin care regimen that targeted her specific skin concerns. Although this incident was many years ago now, as a practicing dermatologist, this memory influences my daily interactions with my patients. At least once a day a patient will come to see me with a large bag of pricey, non-specific products with less-than-desired results. They say, "None of this is working." Alongside my husband, a practicing plastic surgeon, I felt the need to write this book. I want to be able to do for a larger number of people what I was able to do for Claire all those years ago and what I am able to do for my patients each day—to give them a sensible, tailored and realistic plan for their beauty regimen that is based in fact and proven science. My hope is to help cut through the clutter, get down to the basics and help women (and men) make more informed decisions as they explore their health and beauty goals.

When it comes to products that address aging, I see a lot of brands making bold, important strides in this realm of science. From innovative ingredients to bespoke product lines, it's all very exciting. As a woman interested in skin care, there's a lot to love; but as a dermatologist, I have to question their marketing approach. There are some brands that can take their claims a little too far, and that only overwhelms us further. When you're standing in the skin care aisle with a dozen labels claiming some version of "Fountain of Youth," it's only natural to feel skeptical, if not a little overwhelmed. I want to help clarify what all this stuff does for your skin and whether or not you actually need it.

The skin care aisle can feel a little daunting, but I have found that this is truer for my patients who walked into it without a clear skin care goal. Taking care of your skin and feeling confident in how you look shouldn't feel like an impossible task, and understanding your personal goals can help eliminate some of that overwhelming feeling.

Through this book I think we can uncover some truths. There will be some things that are tough to swallow (there is no "facelift in a jar"). But, with some foundational knowledge and some guidance to cut through the clutter, I'll highlight useful insight about skin health, aging, beauty and how to make better decisions in your own best interests.

> *My mission in writing this book—and my focus as a dermatologist—is to help you break through the distractions and find what works for you.*

If you are considering a cosmetic procedure or looking for the best beauty routine, you are inundated with information on the internet, at the department store, on TV, at the drugstore and even from your friends. It is difficult to wade through all that information and get what you need. I researched, wrote and organized this book to help you with skin care, noninvasive in-office options and surgical procedures. My goal is to provide clean information, backed with research, to help you zero in on what products, treatments and procedures are best for you. But what works? Come on already—what really works?

As you're reading this book and uncovering information, I hope I can show you how to ignore the clutter of advertising and sensationalized science, and instead focus on ingredients and results that are best for you in the long haul. I'd like you to find more value in the actual procedures and distinct ingredients than in generalized branding, because a brand name does not mean results.

As professionals in dermatology and plastic surgery, my husband and I are trying to highlight the products and procedures that are proven to work. We want you to feel confident about your cosmetic choices and the professionals who assist you. Whether you're interested in prescription-strength topicals, injections, laser, or surgery, this book is our effort to help people everywhere stop lugging the "bag of products" around and get results.

This book is our hitting pause for you. We're sitting down and taking a moment to clear things up, because you deserve the best information to help you make decisions to reach your beauty and skin care goals.

We better get started. There's a lot of clearing up to do.

Beauty: An Overview

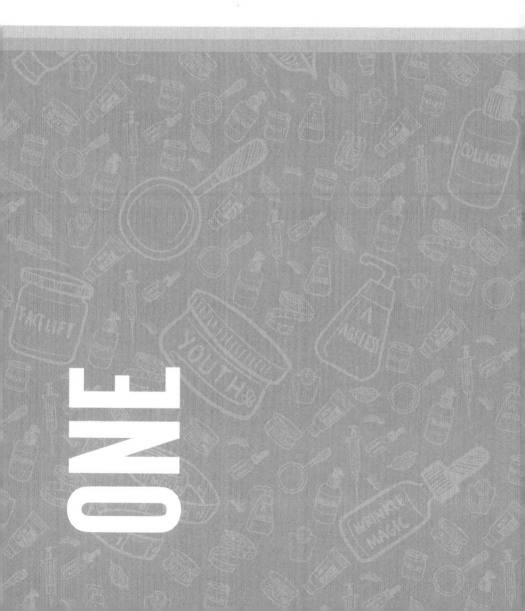

ONE

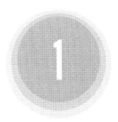

BEAUTY: AN OVERVIEW
WHAT MAKES US BEAUTIFUL?

Is beauty skin deep? Well, if you ask me, as a dermatologist, you might be surprised to hear my answer is … no.

Of course it isn't, because we all have our own perceptions of what is beautiful. Beauty is a complex topic that is both subjective and objective, and our perception of beauty is constructed of perceptions both innate and learned. But this book isn't diving into who is beautiful and who is not. We're talking about the core elements that have historically and scientifically summarized beauty. My medical assistant and patient care coordinator is 60 years old and has been with me for eight years now. During the first few years she worked for me she would share her concerns about small imperfections on her face. I could never see what she was talking about. She finally told me she had been using her 10X magnifying mirror at home—the type that magnifies your face and everything on it. I assured her that she didn't need to waste her worry on imperfections she couldn't even see with a regular mirror and other people definitely couldn't see from five feet away.

When examining our personal beauty, we're often our own worst critics. We have a habit of viewing our faces with a 10X mirror approach, pointing out minor imperfections unnoticeable to the outside person looking in. My job as a dermatologist (and my husband's job as a plastic surgeon) is to help you zoom out so you can see the bigger picture about how you look and how you feel. Part of what helps us do our job well is our deep understanding of beauty from an intellectual standpoint. This is why we need to discuss perceptions of beauty and beauty norms. Outlining beauty standards helps us understand why we value beauty and what drives us to seek improvements in the way we look.

Our value and perception of beauty stems from two factors: innate and learned. Both are equally influential in the way we form impressions of people and how we view beauty in ourselves and in others.

Innate Perception Of Beauty

Our innate concept of beauty is pure impulse, one we are born with, explained by evolutionary psychologists to be an attraction toward healthy humans [1], and therefore someone with whom you would like to mate. (Remember, we are talking about perceptions or impressions here, meaning they are inherently biased.) [2] You've experienced this before. Maybe you've taken in a tropical sunset, a famous painting, or even a stranger walking down the sidewalk, and your breath changed. You felt lighter and fuller all at once. You've witnessed beauty. When we see something or someone beautiful, we feel it first, before we can think about it. That's biological, or innate.

Similarly, caring about our appearance is the result of the innate need to love ourselves and be loved by others. Facial qualities like symmetry, facial averageness (commonness), sexual dimorphism and youthfulness all attribute to a person's inherent attractiveness. [3]

Learned Perception Of Beauty

Our learned perception of beauty is just as it sounds: learned. We adopt perceptions of beauty through cultural standards and through our inner circle's shared perception and looks. Our inner circle usually includes our families and those we grow up around. For example, if your first boyfriend or girlfriend had red hair, it would come as no surprise if you grew up and became attracted to redheads. Studies have also shown we learn to become attracted to people with self-similar features (specifically eye color and hair color) as well as features present in our opposite-sex parent. [4] Personal learned preferences develop early in life, often before cultural standards can influence them. [5]

If beauty is in the eye of the beholder, then in many ways the beholder is the culture in which you associate. Cultural beauty and age standards play a major role in our learned perception of others and ourselves. I see this with my own patients, as does my husband as a plastic surgeon. What they identify as beautiful and what they would like to enhance on their faces and bodies is in line with their culture's standard of beauty. This could mean skin treatments, breast or buttocks augmentation, nose reconstruction, lip filler or any number of things.

In certain cultures in Thailand, women place heavy rings around their neck to achieve an elongated neck. Women in certain regions of Ethiopia intentionally scar their bodies as a sign of sensuality and beauty. Here in America, we're currently fans of full lips and large, shapely behinds. The increase in requests for lip filler and the Brazilian butt lift procedures are testaments to that.

THE CORE ELEMENTS OF BEAUTY

A great deal of our understanding of beauty comes from primal instincts and observations. In this section we've identified our seven core elements of beauty to help you get your arms around the paradigm of beauty in relation to health and vitality.

1. Symmetry
2. Proportion
3. Commonness or being in the "Normal Range"
4. Gender Norms Masculine or Feminine (Sexual Dimorphism)
5. Skin Complexion and Texture
6. Youthfulness
7. Dominant Trait

These seven core elements of beauty are a general reference for medical professionals in cosmetic medicine and do not encompass the largely subjective nature of beauty.

Symmetry
Our attraction to symmetry is undeniable. In fact, it can be considered innate. When someone is looking for an aesthetic improvement, they're

often looking for options that make their features more symmetrical, or as symmetrical as possible. Symmetry is one of the more discussed factors contributing to beauty.

Symmetry, or the appearance of symmetry (since no one has a perfectly symmetrical face), has been proven over and over again to be a primary component in our definition of beauty. We are so attracted to symmetrical faces and bodies that evolutionary psychologists have theorized symmetry might insinuate good health during our early development. [6] According to the perceptual bias theory, symmetry is attractive to us because it is more easily processed by our visual system. [7] While moderately asymmetrical features can certainly be attractive (crooked nose, lone dimples and cocked smiles) in aesthetic medicine, symmetry is a reliable standard we use to improve the overall appeal of the face and body. Rarely, rarely, rarely would someone ever ask to have surgery to make one eyebrow raised a few centimeters higher than the other. Understandably, with our evolutionary, hard-wired attraction to symmetry, patients often request products, treatments and procedures that result in their features appearing more symmetric.

Proportion

Proportion is another element that pleases our innate perception of beauty. Proportion refers to the structure of the face (or body) based on ratio. The distance between the eyes, distance from eyes to mouth, length of the nose and length of the chin all inform the face's relation to the Golden Ratio, or 1:1.618. [8] We have an innate fondness for this ratio. Leonardo da Vinci's famous Vitruvian Man drawings emphasized proportion in both the figure and the face, and the ratio is clear in the Mona Lisa as well. One study used the Golden Ratio as the point of research to determine whether beauty, as a whole, was more objective or subjective (i.e. innate or learned). [9] Researchers had everyday people—meaning those without a specific knowledge or expertise in the arts—look at sculptures as if they were in a museum. Participants showed clear approval and pleasure from sculptures that followed the Golden Ratio. This is just one of several studies identifying the Golden Ratio (and proportion) as a contributing factor to our innate perception of beauty.

For the body, despite how drastically our learned or cultural standard of beauty has appeared to change (from full figured bombshells to stick thin celebrities to muscular, fit bodies) what remains innately attractive is proportion. That is what plastic surgeons can help with. We often have patients with an apple shape come in looking for liposuction in the tummy, so that their top is proportionate to their bottom. Female patients with a pear shape come in to get breast implants so they are more proportionate. Some males are self-conscious of their "stick legs" compared to their filled out chests. While it's less common, some men fix this with calf implants. We like proportionate shapes.

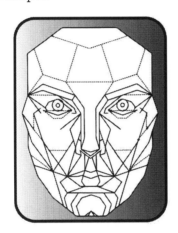

Commonness

Commonness doesn't mean looking like a "Plain Jane." It simply means we are attracted to individuals who are within the population mean or, if you took statistics, within the bell curve of typical human features. [10] I have a patient who uses online dating sites and refuses to put an up-to-date photo of herself on her profile. Her photos portray her as easily 10 years younger than she really is. From my experience, she is not trying to be misleading, she wants to be portrayed on the dating site as her ideal self, as the person she feels that she is.

When patients come to my office, they are often looking to be put back into the "normal range." Sometimes that "normal range" is their age group, sometimes that "normal range" is how they looked 5 years ago or the look that most of their friends have. I hear it all the time:

- I don't want my cheeks looking too big.
- I want to still look like me.
- I just want to look less tired.
- I would be thrilled if I could have the lips I used to have.

Generally, we don't seek out fillers or surgery because we want to look different; we want to look closer to both our personal normal and the norm of our friend group and our cultural group. We want in the box. The pillar of "Commonness" is the idea of this box, composed partly by math like the golden ratio and partly by social standards. Outside of this box is the size of some celebrities' backsides and lips. I rarely have people ask me to make their lips or buttocks that large. Interestingly they often use this as an example of what they don't want. They don't want to be too far out of the "normal range" or box, they want to look like a better version of themselves. Most of us are not consciously aware of how important commonness or being within the box is in overall attractiveness; but haven't most of us discussed or heard it discussed about a celebrity's feature that is out of that box as being extreme or unattractive? We are innately cautious of extreme or out-of-the-box traits in one another because we've evolved to associate them with undesired genetic traits—genes that could be a sign of genetic disorder, disease or weakness. Studies have shown that symmetry and commonness work hand in hand. Together, these two factors help us make impressions about people who are more disease resistant (or more healthy; and therefore, more desirable as a mate because they have "good" genes to pass on to future children). [11]

Feminine and Masculine Features (Sexual Dimorphism)
There are characteristic features that identify female beauty and male handsomeness. We identify with someone as male or female based on these characteristics. From an evolutionary standpoint this admiration for sexual dimorphism is innate in order to find a mate and reproduce.

- **Standard Feminine Attributes** - Characteristic female traits are arched eyebrows, a smooth vertical forehead and a smaller nose. Females also have more fat in their cheeks, making the face fuller. They are softer with less hair on the face and glowing complexions.
- **Standard Masculine Attributes** - Men have more deeply set eyes, larger

noses, flatter eyebrows, a thinner top lip and a strong jawline and chin. Male foreheads are broader and higher than female foreheads. Their foreheads typically have a ridge above the eyes, making their brow line more pronounced. [12]

Why are masculine and feminine traits considered a beauty standard?

We can trace most of these core elements of beauty to our evolutionary or innate impressions of beauty. The indication of beauty we are addressing here is your identification with a gender and the corresponding feminine or masculine traits for that identification. Strong masculine traits indicate "physical fitness" in the evolutionary sense of the term, meaning that person can withstand the stress that high levels of testosterone can put on the body. [13] Strong feminine traits indicate that a person is sexually mature and fertile. These traits connect to the core element of beauty: youth. We typically demonstrate our strongest masculine and feminine traits in our peak fertility years. As we age and our hormone levels begin to shift (first up, then down), it's common to see changes in the face, for better or for worse (aesthetically speaking). For instance, as men lose testosterone, their muscle mass decreases. As women lose estrogen, they begin to shift the way they carry weight from the hip and thigh area to the stomach. Sometimes these hormonal changes can cause aesthetic changes that the patient wants to address. It's common for women to get laser hair removal when they begin seeing stray facial hair on the chin or around the mouth. Men might get injectables or fillers or even a facelift to restore a strong jawline or other typically masculine facial feature.

Again, the relationship between attractiveness and gender is all pretty complex. For example, masculine traits become more attractive to women during times when they are more likely to become pregnant (ovulation) or when they are looking for short-term relationships. [14] This indicates that our personal preferences aren't so black and white and are expected to change under different circumstances.

While hormones can dictate what's characteristically feminine or masculine, what's "beautiful" is determined by our learned personal and cultural standard of beauty. Beauty trends shift, even in what is considered masculine and feminine. In fact we are seeing a shift in the role of masculine/feminine characteristics in beauty today. Androgynous looks are also becoming fashionable again, just as it was in the '60s Twiggy era. We see it booming in the beauty industry (unisex skin care lines, ambiguously sexy hairstyles, clothing lines … the list is long).

I should note that the work I am referring to does not represent or characterize patients seeking gender reassignment surgery, which is entirely different. Patients on the path for gender reassignment surgery are committed to making changes that transcend the aesthetic into the medical and psychological, and their journey through transition as well as their medical support system reflects that. Gender reassignment surgery is a recently much publicized topic. It is interesting to note that during gender reassignment surgery most transitions happen by accentuating the new gender's dominant beauty traits. Look at the famous Caitlyn Jenner. She did not just have breast implants put in to become a woman, she has been very open about the hormone therapy, jaw shaving, rhinoplasty and volume restoration of the face she has received to have a more feminine look. She has moved away from the strong jaw and volume deficient face to the more narrow, sleek jaw with higher cheekbones. Gender reassignment surgery supports the idea that masculinity and femininity are beauty pillars.

Skin Complexion and Texture

Together, skin complexion and texture make up the fifth beauty pillar. Glowing skin and a clear, smooth complexion are a couple of those innate factors of beauty at the top of every man and woman's wish list. In fact good skin is at the cornerstone of the beauty and skin care industry. As a nation, we spend billions of dollars each year on acne solutions, exfoliants, masks, facials and other treatments to achieve our best skin—and that's just skin care! [15] In makeup we have game changing primers, foundations, highlighters and shimmery products to give us that glowing complexion. From an evolutionary perspective, our innate desire for beautiful skin is so strong because it indicates that we could be healthy mates to others. Healthy skin adds to that youthful appearance and vitality we're striving for. While topical treatments and makeup are indeed essential to beautiful skin, a good complexion is part genetics, part environment, part nutrition and part hormonal. Your complexion is an indicator of your overall health to the outside observer, and health is a major underlying factor of this pillar of beauty.

Youth and Fertility

Quick, think of someone you'd consider a beauty icon. Did you picture a Hollywood star in his or her 20s or 30s? I thought Cindy Crawford, but as her 20-year-old self (even though she is still drop dead gorgeous!). That's not surprising. Even beauty icons from 70 years ago are usually remembered by portraits from their 20s or 30s. The logic is innate. Youth flaunts robust reproductive traits. Cheeks are plump and supple, frames are proportionate and fat layers and muscle tissues are propping everything up just right. See, in your 20s and 30s, you're ripe for reproduction, rendering you more attractive in a primal sort of way. Both societal standards and biological impulses have ranked youth as a vital component of what makes someone beautiful.

Ready for the great news? With proper at home care and help from your dermatologist, you can boast a youthful appearance for decades after 30. I'm not talking about magic either. While eating right, hydrating and sleeping will always be part of creating a youthful appearance (I can't stress that enough), once you start coming across stubborn fine lines, fat pockets or drooping, a little help can go a long way.

Dominant Feature

Everybody has a dominant feature—red hair, bushy eyebrows, or a roman nose, to name a few. Some people accentuate it. Cindy Crawford, Madonna and Sofia Loren were all known for their beauty marks, for example. Of course once they embraced their beauty marks, the look quickly became trendy. I remember people drawing in beauty marks for a whole decade. In fact, it seems celebrities are far more likely to embrace their dominant feature and establish it as their signature look. Consider supermodels Lauren Hutton and Lara Stone who kept their gap teeth. Lopez, Beyoncé and the Kardashians brought back the "booty." Once it becomes a signature look to the celebrity, it trickles down into the mainstream of what's within the norm today.

A common dominant feature for many people is the size of their nose. My husband, Dr. Timothy Janiga often takes the bump off of Roman noses and reshapes hooknoses because patients want a nose that doesn't dominate their face. No matter what the dominant feature is—nose, eyebrows, lips and forehead—it is common for people to want to move closer to the middle. Plastic surgeons are able to use standards like the Golden Ratio to reshape noses and improve proportions for a more attractive portrait. I once had a patient who had a broad nose that he thought was wide and unfriendly. He saw my husband for a consultation and he chose to have it reshaped to be closer to the "normal range." After surgery, he told us that he felt like he had a "friendlier" nose and that complete strangers have started smiling at him since the surgery. Did he now get smiles because he was more confident or was his nose really friendlier?

The dominant features we're given at birth are typically separate from the dominant aging feature we acquire as we age. Some people see sagging in the neckline, others see deep wrinkles around the eyes, and others get age spots first. When we evaluate aging, we can address this dominant aging feature first to make the most improvement for our patient.

The Relationship Between Beauty and Aging

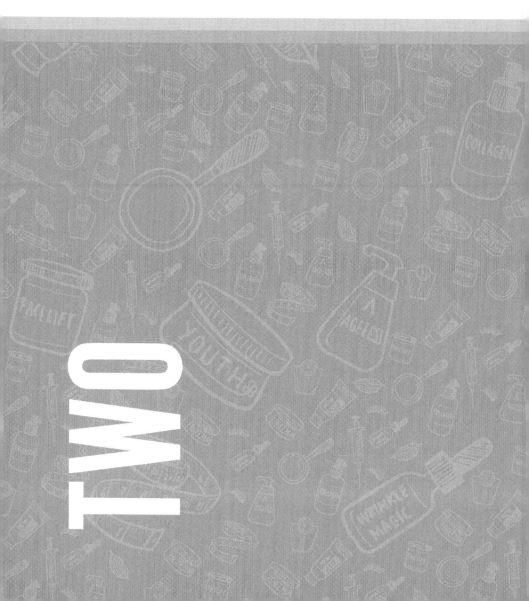

TWO

THE RELATIONSHIP BETWEEN BEAUTY AND AGING

Have you ever heard that saying, "You don't stop having fun because you get old, you get old because you stop having fun," or simply, "You're only as old as you feel"? I think there's quite a bit of truth to these timeless sayings. To feel young, act young and smile, is to look young. In this way, beauty is skin deep if you believe it is.

There is a strong and undeniable connection between how we feel and how we look. Some of our older patients come in bright and unaffected by certain inevitabilities of aging. They embrace them. Other patients feel held back by certain physical indications of aging. Just looking at certain wrinkles makes them feel older all over, and this is what they portray to the world.

While research on this is still in its infancy, there are studies that indicate a connection between how old you feel and how old you look. [1] I personally think laughter, smiling and having a sense of humor are a huge part of what keeps people feeling, and in turn, looking, younger. In fact, laughter therapy has recently been shown to improve vitality in the elderly. [2] Think of Betty White. At the time I'm writing this book, she is 95 years old, and she still has that sparkle in her eye and a huge smile. Has she also taken steps to enhance her health and beauty? I don't know, but I want some of the sparkle.

In cosmetic medicine we are experts in the relationship between beauty and aging, providing treatments and procedures to improve appearance, as we most commonly associate beauty with youth and vitality. If we look back to the sixth pillar of beauty, Youth and Fertility, these characteristics are innately associated with beauty because we find fertility beautiful. Age, however isn't directly aligned with beauty, as physical age and chronological age are not necessarily the same thing. Physical age is the age others perceive us to be because of physical signs of the aging process; whereas Chronologic age is the actual number of years we've lived. Physical aging can be controlled (to an extent), while chronological aging cannot. In my practice I have 3D models, photos, books, and even a slide presentation to help my patients understand the changes that come with aging. We discuss the history, genetics, evolution and chronicity in order to better understand what is happening. Once we understand these things we make better choices about how and what things we would like to improve upon.

Our experience with chronologically older people is still pretty new. The average lifespan of a human being is about 80 years old, while 100 years ago it was about half that. [3] In the early 1900s, most men and women died young, like plump grapes, never aging into raisins. Because of the lower average lifespan, we've only been researching aging and what it does to the elderly body for about a century. For women, life expectancy passed into the 70s in the 1950s, and this was the time when people by and large started to regularly see what an "older woman" looked like. It was different and unfamiliar, and so the treatment of aging took off. Therefore, the treatment of aging as we know it hasn't even reached 70 years old. Most of what we know has been discovered only recently, and there is much more to come. Technology in cosmetic and medical industries is advancing rapidly.

Age is Just a Number: Factors that Influence Signs of Aging

We all age, but we have some control over how fast we show our age. Some people look 5-10 years younger than their age; others look 5-10 years older. Some of this is because of genetics—things like dark circles, dominant features and certain skin conditions. Aside from that, there are some methods for optimizing the hand you're dealt. Factors like diet, sleep, sun protection and exercise can (and should) be managed if you want to maintain a youthful appearance.

A major part of graceful aging is how you take care of your body. After all, modern medicine admits there is only so much we can do with a cream, a syringe or in the operating room. Everything we put in our bodies and expose it to has a role in how we age. It's not the sexiest advice, but taking good care of yourself can help you live a life of graceful aging. Have I always done everything correctly? No. When I was seventeen I was a lifeguard. Sunscreen as we know it today was barely getting a start. The only thing I had access to was SPF 4. I spent my lifeguard days baking under the desert sun—not ideal for skin care. I also went to college in San Diego and spent many a Sunday afternoon on the beach. We now have options for sunscreen and information about sun and aging to help us make better decisions. I would like to think my seventeen-year-old self would do better if she knew better; but then again, how many savvy 17-year-olds do you know?

Below I have identified a few main factors that contribute to the appearance of aging. I should note these factors do not exist in silos. All of these factors can be interconnected through lifestyle choices. Stress, for example, is known to affect sleep patterns. Stress also contributes to occasional excessive drinking, smoking and consumption of unhealthy foods. The good news is, significantly reducing even one of these factors will likely lead to a domino effect.

Smoking

Smoking cigarettes is a major skin offender, as it weakens and destroys the components of the skin that contribute to a youthful impression. This causes the skin to look older before its time. Tobacco contains thousands of chemicals (many of which are carcinogenic) that damage the skin both inside and out. Cigarette smoke is a toxin that constricts the blood vessels and deprives the skin of blood supply. Smokers tend to have a yellowing of the skin around the mouth, uneven skin tone, and develop lines around the mouth and on the lips. In addition, the toxins themselves damage the skin directly. These chemicals damage elastin and collagen in the skin. A recent twin study examined skin aging between twins at the Twins Day Festival in Twinsburg, Ohio. Researchers identified and photographed twins who had different smoking history. The difference in the twins' complexion, texture, color, laxity and other signs of aging was astonishing. The study showed the twins that smoked had a physical age of about 2.5 years older than the twin counterparts that did not smoke. [4]

Stress

Our skin has long been identified as a stage for signs of both acute and chronic stress in the body. [5] As our largest organ, it is a primary communicator of our overall health, reacting to external stressors and also demonstrating some of these stress responses on the skin. Stress is associated with certain chemicals in our bodies—Cortisol, Norepinephrine and Adrenaline, to name a few. These "stress chemicals" help us cope with stress in sudden, small doses (like when we are being chased by a bear); but if we become chronically stressed and these chemicals are continually produced, they can lead to premature aging. Chronic stress damages cells and shortens the DNA telomeres (the areas at the end of our chromosomes that fuse with neighboring chromosomes). Cortisol hardens arteries and lowers growth hormones. Since chronic stress lowers the skin's immunity, high cortisol levels can accelerate signs of aging like fine lines, wrinkles and dull, saggy skin. [6] Norepinephrine speeds up our heart rate and interferes with our ability to focus. Adrenaline, or more famously known as the fight-or-flight hormone, also speeds up our heart rate and compromises digestion, keeping us from absorbing beneficial nutrients from our food.

There is a connection between acute stress and insomnia as well as depression, which both have their own hand in increasing the appearance of aging. [7]

Sugary Diet

For your diet I offer two mantras: "Let food be your medicine," and "Preservatives in your food do not preserve your body." Your diet dictates the production and protection of important building blocks in your organs, including your skin and other tissues.

You are likely aware that the average American diet is overrun with high-calorie, processed foods, which have contributed to the rise of diabetes, heart disease and obesity. These foods also cause high levels of insulin in your bloodstream, which accelerates wrinkling in the skin. The best possible method for protecting your body from aging is through a diet filled with whole fresh foods, leafy greens, lean proteins and "good" fats, also known as unsaturated fats.

When you eat sugar, the molecule latches onto the skin-firming proteins in your bloodstream, a process called glycation. [8] Together, the protein and sugars create a harmful molecule called advanced glycation end products or, ironically enough, AGEs for short. The more sugar you consume, the more AGEs accumulate in the body, causing disruption and the skin barrier and accelerated aging.

Unfortunately, you cannot use artificial sugars as a workaround, either. Artificial sweeteners such as aspartame have no nutritional value and can cause inflammation in the body, a known culprit of accelerated aging. Artificial sweeteners also train our bodies to crave other sweet foods therefore actually increasing calorie consumption. [9] The American Journal of Clinical Nutrition warns that processed sugars trigger the release of inflammatory messengers called cytokines.

In the bigger picture, my philosophy is that most things in moderation are fine (except smoking and drugs). When I say moderation I'm talking about a piece of dark chocolate, missing sleep for a few nights to take care of a sick friend, or going on a cleanse for a few days to lose a little holiday weight. If you are worried about glycation from sugar, and you are following the concept of the bigger picture healthy diet, stop stressing (that ages you, too!). You are probably doing just fine.

However, if your diet consists mainly of sugar and processed foods, and you find that you're 30 pounds overweight or diabetic, the wrinkles that are being caused by the glycation are second to the overall damage these foods are doing to your whole body. Focusing on overall health will reduce the risks of these health issues and improve signs of aging as well.

While dietary supplements can help you fill in nutritional gaps in your diet, nutrients are most effective when you get them from your food. [10] Plus, too much of any nutrient can actually become harmful. An overdose of vitamin A, for example, can lead to fatal toxicity. Most vitamins have a toxic dose like this. On the other hand, some of the most common vitamin deficiencies are in vitamin D, iron and calcium. If you have deficiencies in any of these, I encourage you to speak to your primary care doctor to make sure you do not have an underlying illness that needs to be treated. Together you can discuss the possibility of supplements if you cannot increase your intake of these vitamins and minerals with your diet. Insert a visual table of important, skin loving and anti-aging nutrients.

The Janiga Health "Rules"

People often ask me what diet my husband and I follow and I used to be hesitant to answer this question because each person is different and what works for one person does not necessarily work for the other. Though, as we have arrived at our mid-forties and have the same pressures of eating healthy while balancing our kids' activities, work, and exercise, I have realized my fellow mid-lifers are not asking about quick fix weight loss diets; they are asking about healthy living diets—long term solutions, not short term ones. With this in mind I will tell you first that I sometimes have ice cream with my kids, some candy at Halloween and cheesecake a couple of times a year. But, more than 90 to 95 percent of the time we eat what I consider whole foods—things that would spoil if you left them out for a few days. For breakfast we usually have eggs or a homemade spinach and fruit smoothie. For lunch we have fruit and some type of lean meat, and dinner is typically salad and or another vegetable and meat. Here and there we may have a little corn, a little potato, and a little rice; but overall we have very little bread, processed food or frozen high sodium meals. We try most things in moderation (have you seen the pattern?). A little ice cream will not harm you, but, in my opinion, a lot will. People will disagree with me about the corn or the rice or even the ice cream and that is fine. This is my philosophy.

Alcohol

Alcohol is a bit controversial in the realm of health and aging. Some research suggests mild to moderate amounts of alcohol may have a protective effect on cholesterol levels, heart disease and stroke (again, everything in moderation!). [11] Moderate consumption is defined as less than one serving for women and two servings for men under 65. A serving is 5 ounces of wine, 12 ounces of beer, or 1.5 ounces of hard liquor. What are absolute are the damaging effects of excess alcohol consumption. If you consume enough alcohol to start damaging your liver it has dehydrating and inflammatory properties. Dehydration makes the signs of aging like fine lines and wrinkles look worse, while inflammation can causes redness of the skin and damage collagen and elastin. Additional research has shown how chronic, excessive alcohol consumption depletes vitamin A (retinoids). [12]

However (and good news!) not all alcohol treats the body in the same way. Red wine supplies the body with polyphenols, a protective antioxidant. [13] That being said, according to the Mayo Clinic, red wine has not been specifically shown to be better for you than other forms of alcohol. But, because hard alcohol is usually consumed with sugary mixers or sugar drinks, this becomes an inflammatory, high calorie drink—a double whammy.

So if alcohol in moderation is ok, am I giving everyone full license to have 1-2 glasses a night? Technically no. Each person's ability to consume alcohol is different and you should take this into consideration. Some people tolerate two servings, while others may only tolerate half a serving. Other things to consider: Alcohol can affect your sleep cycles, increase appetite, and increase urges to smoke, so monitor how alcohol affects your entire health, not just this one area. If you are drinking solely for the antioxidants, spinach is still better for you. If you are drinking for the heart or stroke benefits please discuss this with your doctor, as there may be better ways to protect yourself. If you enjoy a glass of wine a couple of nights a week, as a social activity this is relatively OK.

Sleep Deprivation
Getting your beauty sleep is no fairytale. Skimping on sleep is scientifically proven to be detrimental to beauty. After a poor night's sleep, you might notice dark circles under your eyes, dull complexion and coworkers keep asking, "Are you OK?"

The Center For Disease Control and Prevention reports about 35 percent of Americans regularly sleep less than 7 hours in a given 24-hour period[14]. One study found that over time sleep deprivation can disrupt skin function leading to fine lines, age spots and a weaker ability to recover from sun damage overnight. [15] Chronic sleep deprivation depresses immune function and increases risk of disease.

There are so many reasons why sleep evades us. Certain medications, diet pills and stress all contribute to insomnia, so we take sleeping pills to get to sleep and drink coffee to handle the grogginess; and yet in this cycle we don't have time for what I consider the best method for a good night's sleep: exercise. I cannot emphasize enough how firmly I believe that exercise is the key to a great wake-and-sleep cycle. I recently saw a patient suffering with sleep apnea. He couldn't sleep and claims he has no energy to exercise because of this. Because he is a long-time patient of mine, we have a more open relationship and he welcomes my candor. I pointed out to him that if he reached part of his weight loss goal (which is about 75 pounds) he will likely sleep better, since weight is a significant contributor to sleep apnea. This is a classic chicken and egg scenario. He can't sleep because he cannot exercise, and he cannot exercise because he cannot sleep. I advised him to take his next best day and make a change. (I didn't suggest starting the next day, because some days are better than others, and tomorrow could be the worst day to start something new. That's life, so when I am trying to start a new good habit I pick the next best day and get to it.) Adding 30 minutes of exercise most days can help him get the weight off. Since our conversation he has been doing well and is 50 pounds to his goal. My point in sharing this is to emphasize that sometimes we need to pause in our hectic cycles, look for patterns and get back to the basics. If you want to look younger, feel better, and sleep well, put some emphasis in your life on working out.

Disease
Certain diseases, such as cancer, diabetes, alcoholism and chronic depression, leach the youth right out of us. Our bodies work hard to fight disease, causing our cells to work harder. Certain medical treatments, like chemotherapy, also accelerate aging by killing both good and bad tissue with the primary goal of killing the disease. Disease is categorized as either acute or chronic:

A virus, infection or injury that triggers the body to temporarily overwork the immune system often causes acute disease. These include bacterial or viral infections. Chronic disease has recently been linked to accelerated aging. [16] Chronic diseases often come on slowly, because of poor health habits, genetics or environmental factors. Major Depressive Disorder (MDD), considered a mental illness, causes psychological stress, which stimulate stress-related aging. [17]

Some disease is out of our control and we need to get treatment and get back to our recovery after. There is no sugar coating that. But, some diseases are manageable to an extent and we should seek help as soon as possible to help us be in charge of our own condition.

Hormones
It probably comes as no surprise that hormones are linked to signs of aging. Both men and women have a balance of estrogen and testosterone in their bodies, and this balance shifts as we hit middle age. As men get older they lose testosterone, and as women get older they lose estrogen and progesterone. For women this experience is called Menopause, an accelerated loss of estrogen that occurs as early as our 40s and into our 50s. As a result, collagen production slows. Since this hormone is naturally anti-inflammatory, inflammation, aging, and certain illnesses can increase.

As a young woman my mom always had really great cholesterol levels without a high HDL (good cholesterol) and low LDL (bad cholesterol). She went in to see her doctor in her 50s and her cholesterol had increased significantly and it was now above normal range. She was quite upset to learn this and couldn't figure out what she had done "wrong." But, as it turns out, that was the year she had completed menopause and no longer had her estrogens. Estrogens are protective against cholesterol elevation. She said, "Well how come no one told me that was going to happen?"

Would she have just wondered if her daughter wasn't a doctor and able to help explain it to her; or would she have gone and talk to her physician and found out? I don't know, but education is a powerful tool and knowing what to expect with aging is going to put you ahead of the curve.

As the balance of estrogen and testosterone shifts in women, androgenic characteristics like increased facial hair production and change in body shape can also occur. [18] Women's skin also gets thin, pale, and dry because of this decrease in estrogen. Men and women also lose growth hormone as we get older, which causes more fat deposition, less muscle mass, cells to stop multiplying and our skin to begin sagging. [19] I call the changes that happen to the female body from these changes in growth hormone and estrogen the "mid-life widening." This means the natural hourglass shape most women have before 35, widens in the stomach area to be more of an apple shape. With this decrease in hormones and "mid-life widening," it is common to experience increases in weight, diabetes and cholesterol. So, what can be done to increase growth hormones in your body as you age? The two things that have been proven to increase growth hormone are exercise and sleep. [20] Recent studies have shown men don't slide through middle age so easily either. In addition to the growth hormone decreasing, we have already discussed the male counterpart to female menopause, or andropause, which describes the steady loss in testosterone as men age. While not all men experience symptoms of andropause, those who do may lose muscle mass, increase fat levels and experience erectile dysfunction.

So you ask, "Can I just take growth hormone and estrogen or testosterone in pill or shot form as I age to stay young?" This is not an answer I can quickly give you in a book. The use of supplemental hormones should be discussed with your doctor directly and should be based on your specific risks and other medical conditions. This is a controversial subject and should be based on your specific health history, symptoms and risk to benefit ratio.

Environment

We all have sun-damaged skin unless we have spent our entire lives indoors. It's to what extent and how visible the changes are that concern us cosmetically. Photoaging, or sun damage from ultraviolet rays, causes age spots, wrinkles and damage to the collagen and elastin fibers in the skin. Chronic sun damage leads to mottled pigmentation, dull, sagging skin and even cobblestoning. Think about Magda from Something About Mary. She manifested all of these changes.

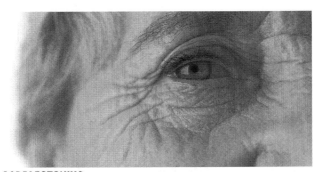

COBBLESTONING

Can Aging Be Reversed?

We frequently hear about new products and treatments that can "reverse" aging, but it's important to understand what qualifies as reversal and what qualifies as superficial improvements. The word "reverse" in aging should refer to deep, cellular change in the tissue where you will have a measurable endpoint response, as opposed to a temporary improvement in aesthetics. If you have a superficial chemical peel for example, you aren't doing much on a cellular level, but it does exfoliate the skin and help your products penetrate better and make your makeup lay nicer on your face. To improve things on a cellular level and by definition then "reverse aging," there are products and procedures that are shown to change the body on a chemical level. Products and procedures that have been scientifically proven to affect change include retinoid, peptides, antioxidants, lasers and growth factors.

Besides the products and procedures known to cause chemical changes, there are some products that can be used preventatively to help prevent the signs of aging. Neuromodulators like BOTOX® and Dysport® are continuing to increase in popularity for this reason, among others. Long term, consistent application of these neuromodulators relaxes the muscles and prevents expression lines from forming. The science behind this is straightforward: if the lines never form, then you do not have to try to reverse them later.

In my research and experience you can see a significant difference between people who worked outdoor jobs for the past 20 years and those with indoor jobs. This difference is most noticeable in people that live in sunny climates or high elevations. It is less noticeable in cloudy climates like England. Most 40-year-olds who have appropriately protected their skin from the sun appear younger than their stated age. [21]

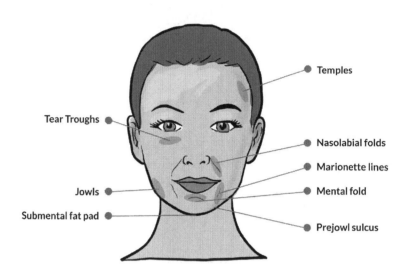

The Aging Face and Body

Beauty might not be skin deep, but physical aging is closer to it. (Technically, aging is bone deep). Physical aging is a tricky thing. You might feel 25, but when you look in the mirror and see lines and colors that don't belong there, you can't help but think the vitality you feel inside is not what other people see on the outside. While there's something to be said for embracing signs of aging, by no means do we need to embrace every age spot and wrinkle. Science allows us to close the gap between how old we look and how young we feel.

Your skin is a great indicator of overall wellness. You know when you're dehydrated when your lips are dry, and you know to expect some dark circles under your eyes after a poor night's sleep (or a long night out). Over time, and as early as your 20s, these hints for your health settle in for good, although it can feel like you've aged overnight. Common signs of aging are accelerated by unhealthy lifestyle choices, so the earlier you can start wearing sunscreen, eating, sleeping and exercising regularly, the better you will look after 40.

If you're like most of us, you feel you've done (mostly) everything right, but despite your best efforts those wrinkles, brown spots and crepey skin are creeping up on you. In order to make the outside of you reflect how you feel inside, you might be tempted to dump the whole anti-aging aisle into your cart, or maybe you want to get a full facelift. While both are options, it's possible neither will be a good fit for your specific signs of aging. I consult patients every day who come in wanting a specific procedure or product to help their skin, but they actually need a completely different plan than they were asking for. But what is happening deep beneath the surface to cause wrinkles, hollowness, spots and other unwanted signs? To understand aging, we have to look deeper to see what's going on at each level; we have to understand what's happening in our bones. So, let's talk about the levels of physical aging, from the surface of the skin down to the bone level. This will help you as the consumer understand the process of aging better. In these next sections, we'll look at a few different factors to determine physical age.

Facial aging and body aging are similar but distinct processes. Let's discuss these changes that contribute to the aging process, from the inside out.

Bone Density and Volume Loss

Most of us reach our peak bone mass around age 30, and from there we experience a gradual decline in bone density and volume. The bones of the face are no different. The facial skeleton experiences an overall decrease in volume and projection, or what is called morphologic change. This bone loss causes our temples to narrow, our cheeks to become less prominent, our eyes to look more hallow, and the jawline to retract. This is why most men and women over the age of 80 have the similar look of a small mouth that appears almost inverted. It is partly the loss of bone structure in the face.

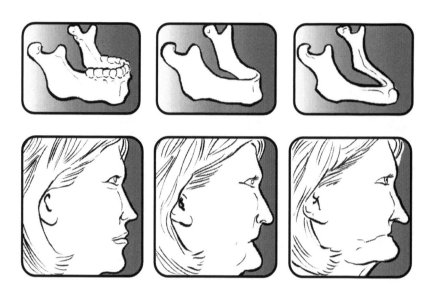

In a study comparing the skulls of 18-30-year-olds to the skulls of 55-65-year-olds, the skull shape and structure difference is amazing. In the younger face there is more projection of the forehead and cheekbones while in an older face there is loss in the projection. [22] In addition, the angles of the facial bones change. As the bones in the body age and become more brittle, the jawbone also thins and becomes less defined. The orbital rim of the eyeball sinks in and becomes long and thin. All of this results in less support for the skin and soft tissue on top, which manifests as jowling of the skin or laxity.

To augment the contours of the bones that have lost projection and density with the aging process, we use your own tissue or implants to rebalance the face to more youthful proportions. Implants can be silicone solid implants, fat or fillers like Juvéderm®, Restylane®, Radiesse® or Sculptra®. At times your own tissue can be used by surgical correction of the jaw line or even your own taken from a different location such as the abdomen to improve areas that are deficient. Silicone solid implants are placed surgically by a plastic surgeon to improve projection of the cheeks or chin. Fillers are the other type of implantable. Fillers come in many different forms and are FDA approved for different areas. In this section we are specifically discussing the ones that can be placed deep to improve boney projection, but there are many fillers on the market for different purposes. To use your own tissue for improvement of projection is also a possibility. Chin augmentation can sometimes be performed with your own tissue and a surgical plate, but you will need to discuss this with a board-certified plastic surgeon who will examine you and see if this is an option for you. You can also use your own fat. It is harvested by liposuction from another area and placed in the desired area of augmentation.

Muscle Sagging and Cartilage Reduction

Like the bones that lose volume and projection, other tissues in the face and body contribute to the signs of aging. In our 30s we begin to lose lean body mass, and the muscles become less defined. The superficial muscular aponeurotic system (SMAS), which is an extension of the muscles of the face, more or less envelops the facial muscles. The SMAS, like other muscles in the body, becomes less robust and weakens with age. The muscle gets lax in the face, causing that sagging look in the neck and jawline. This is where a facelift can help. The SMAS also loses elasticity, contributing to those fine lines and wrinkles caused by repeated motions, like wrinkling your nose or furrowing your brow. Injectables like BOTOX® can help smooth out these expression lines.

Cartilage in the nose may droop as the connective tissue weakens. This is the reason we have the thought that our nose and ears get larger as we age, when in fact it is the cartilage falling in reaction to gravity. That, coupled with decreasing volume in the face, makes your nose and ears look much larger or like they have grown with age.

If you're my age you likely have heard the phrase "long in the tooth," which refers to the signs of aging that occur to the tissue inside our mouths, mainly the gums. While the tissue inside your mouth is notably resilient, signs of aging occur over time. When you're young, you have nice, beefy gums. But as we age, we lose support structure and volume once provided by those beefy gums, known as the gingiva. Your gums are composed of mucosal tissue that recedes with time. In extreme (though common) cases, receding can lead to periodontal disease. This is why most women over 80 appear as if they have no teeth and most 20-somethings have a nice slope to the upper lip. The slope is being held up and out by their young and full gums, teeth and jawbone.

About That Jaw Device Infomercial ...

I have seen a few infomercials for devices that help exercise the jaw muscles to improve its shape. Like exercise other places, stimulating the muscle can increase volume of the muscle, like building your biceps; but this will not "lift" your face, it will at best increase the muscle in that area to be bulkier.

Fat Drifting and Volume Loss

We all have fat pads on top of muscle and below the skin, and some of those pads weave into the muscle. Think of the fat pads as puzzle pieces under the skin that fit together nicely in your youth and then start to float apart and shrink as you age. This subcutaneous (which means "situated under the skin") fat layer acts as the foundation for your skin, giving your face and neck that smooth and supple look during your youth. This fat layer is like the foundation of a building. When it's new and solid, the building stands upright with every beam and wall right where it should be (this helps create the triangle of youth, which we discuss in depth in the section *Put Your Money Where Your Face Is: Special Considerations for Your Face, Neck and Chest*). Over time, this foundation begins to shrink and fall, which causes the outer layers of skin and facial features to adjust ... sink, wrinkle and sag. In our 20s, our face is voluminous on the upper third, and as we age, those fat pads shrink and fall so the upper third appears hollow and the lower two-thirds of the face look fuller, changing the proportions of the face from a youthful upside-down triangle to more of a rounded oval.

Subcutaneous aging occurs differently for each person. The loss of the fat layer occurs naturally with age but can also occur if you lose weight. If you've ever considered someone as baby face, they probably have a rounder, fuller youthful face. Lucky them! If you have more volume in your face from the start, you are likely to look younger for longer, at least where volume is concerned. Recently I lost 10 pounds and immediately saw a difference in my face. It looked more hollow, angular and long. My weight loss was a decision to better my health, but I didn't want to look older because of it, so I replaced some of the volume I lost with that 10 pounds with some filler into my temples, cheeks and tear trough.

Skin Aging

Skin is usually the first place we notice signs of aging. In your 30s your skin starts to thin; the elastin and collagen break down more rapidly and your skin might start looking a little drier. Since the skin under your eyes is already so thin, it may thin there first. You may notice the first brown spot or broken blood vessel, or the start of fine lines around the eyes or between the brows may begin. Each person ages differently. For me, the first sign was horizontal lines on my forehead. By your 40s, turnover of the skin slows down significantly, and can cause a loss of brightness of the skin. You lose about 1-3 percent of your collagen each year after age 30, so you may start to see some laxity starting or new lines around the eyes. Into the 50s and 60s you will notice the most drying of the skin because of the accumulation of all the things we have discussed but in addition this is the time when our hormones begin to really decrease which compounds the dryness. The cumulative sun damage may show up with significant color changes on the skin as well as collagen breakdown and deeper lines.

As a dermatologist the skin is my domain. The lines, brown spots, dullness, sagging and dryness are some of the most common reasons that people come to see me. But, as you have seen already in this book, the skin signs are usually connected to the underlying structures, so many times the full process requires a combined approach between my husband and myself to get the patient their best result.

At most layers of tissue, you have options for improving signs of aging, though it might not be immediately obvious which cream or procedure is appropriate for you. For instance, you might have done a great job throughout your life protecting your skin, so you don't have sunspots, but you might start to notice a significant volume loss in your face. In these situations, it is up to both you and your medical practitioner to explore options and decide on the proper treatment, if this bothers you.

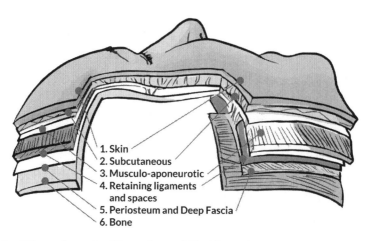

1. Skin
2. Subcutaneous
3. Musculo-aponeurotic
4. Retaining ligaments and spaces
5. Periosteum and Deep Fascia
6. Bone

Our Skin: Hypodermis, Dermis and Epidermis

Despite examining, touching, and assessing our skin, the science of aging is in its infancy and the cellular changes are much more intricate and involved than what we can understand, see or touch. While aging is an undeniable part of life, as the technology of cosmetic procedures and cosmetic topical treatments continue to advance, there is a way to improve, prevent and treat the signs of aging in the skin. There are many products and procedures that help you slow down your skin's aging process (and I promise we are going to go through them). Before you can select the right treatments and procedures, you have to know what type of skin and options for your skin you're working with. As you probably know, your skin is your biggest organ, tasked with the vital role of being the barrier to the outside world. The skin protects your insides from the environment and manages what goes in and out of your system. The skin has three main layers, the epidermis, the dermis and the hypodermis, all of which are affected by aging.

Epidermis and Cell Turnover

The top most layer of your skin showcases the most skin damage. The top layer of the epidermis, called the stratum corneum, used to be considered just a layer of dead cells. Now we know that the stratum corneum is a dynamic and active tissue that has an array of molecules that manage water and exfoliation. When it is able to maintain its balance, it is a flexible and smooth system that looks soft and supple. We are constantly turning over our skin, but as we get older the skin cell turnover slows down causing skin cells to build up. This buildup causes the skin to lose its lustrous, moist traits and appear dull and flaky over time. Retinoid treatments can improve the cell turn over at the deepest levels and exfoliation can help keep the superficial epidermal cells to look smooth.

The deeper layer of the epidermis contains basal cells, which make new cells: immune cells to fight infection and melanocytes, or the cells that make pigment. All of these functions can become less efficient as you age.

Dermis and Collagen

Below the epidermis sits the dermis, a thick layer made up of those favorite youth components we have been talking about called collagen, elastin and hyaluronic acid. The dermis also contains hair follicles, sweat glands, sebaceous glands, nerves, blood vessel connections and collagen and elastin producing fibroblasts.

We have the most collagen production when we're children, and it slows down during our teen years and more dramatically in our 30s and 40s, when we begin to actually lose 1 to 3 percent of our collagen per year. This is why you begin to see signs of aging during these years. Imagine that it's thick and robust in youth and becomes thin and fibular over time, causing wisps of degradation. This degrading of collagen is because of collagenase, a vital enzyme in our skin needed for scar healing that helps remodel the scar tissue. Although, the irony of collagenase is that it's the same enzyme that degrades all collagen over time, giving us those signs of laxity.

Aging isn't only caused by how much or how little collagen we have, but also the quality of collagen in the dermis. The skin—including the vital components of collagen, elastin and hyaluronic acid—is in a necessary and constant cycle of repair and regeneration. As we get older their production decreases. Aging and sun exposure damage the collagen, elastin and hyaluronic acid in the skin, which causes the skin to look more wrinkled, dry and saggy. The good news is a lot of these concerns can be treated with procedures like lasers and chemical peels. We will talk more about this later in the Topical Essentials section.

Subcutaneous Tissue and Hypodermis

The thick, fatty deepest layer of the skin is called the hypodermis, or the subcutaneous fat layer. It attaches your skin to the underlying structures, houses blood vessels and nerves that go from the skin to the rest of the body, helps control body temperature and makes up the fat layer below the skin.

The hypodermis is primarily a fat layer. Fat is technically a loose connective tissue, and it acts as a protective barrier to the muscle and bone. In your youth, this fat layer is present despite your size. You can be at a normal weight by all accounts, but you still have thicker fat layer protecting you when you are young. The dermis and the fat layer work in the same way on both our face and body, until we age and those tissue decrease. Older women come in and say, "I bruise on my arms now. I never used to bruise. What's happened?" You've lost collagen, elastin and the fat layer that was cushioning those blood vessels. In addition, the walls of those vessels have become more friable with chronic sun damage. Now they are more exposed and more easily traumatized, leading to bruising.

As we've seen the production of collagen, elastin, and hyaluronic acid decrease, water transfer to the epidermis decreases, cell turnover decreases, fat cells shrink and a decrease in estrogen thins and dries out the skin as we age. Ooph. So, what can we do about it? The good news: topical preparations and cosmetic treatments we use today can postpone, halt and improve the appearance of these signs of aging!

 Are You and Your Skin the Same Age?

The age of our skin isn't always the same as our actual age. I'm sure you've met people that look 10 years younger than their age and vice versa. Knowing how old your skin is can help you choose treatments and products that are better suited for your needs.

QUIZ

1. **Skin Texture**

    a.   Smooth and supple

    b.   Mostly smooth, but with some dry spots

    c.   Uneven, dry with some flakey spots

    d.   Thing, dry and flakey with some sagging

    e.   Dry, crepe-like with sagging and wrinkles

2. **Skin Tone**

    a.   Even skin tone, glowing

    b.   Mostly glowing, mild discoloration from sun exposure

    c.   Still radiant, though now with moderate discoloration and age spots

    d.   Dull, blotchy, uneven skin tone with clear age spots

    e.   Dull, yellowish tone with pasty complexion and age spots

3. **Fine Lines and Wrinkles**

    a.   Few, if any fine lines

    b.   Faint lines between the eyebrows or around the eyes

    c.   Lines in the forehead or around the eyes when face is relaxed

    d.   Deeper line around the eyes, on the forehead and around the mouth

    e.   Everything in "D" plus deep wrinkles in the cheeks and upper lips

RESULTS

Mostly A – 20s

Mostly B – 30s

Mostly C – 40s

Mostly D – 50s

Mostly E – 60s

If you are looking for a more comprehensive test, there are also apps like the one from Olay® that can help guide you. I think most of us know if we have significant photo aging compared to our friends, but these tests and apps are a fun way of investigating and beginning to engage in your skin health.

Knowing Your Skin Type

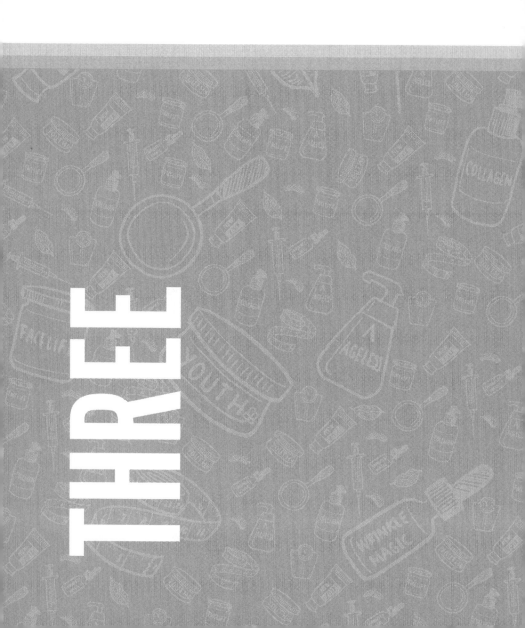

THREE

3

KNOWING YOUR SKIN TYPE

Each person ages in a way that is totally unique to them, based on skin type, skin classification, genetics and lifestyle. As topical skin care brands continue to advance and become more customized to the individual, knowing what your skin actually needs and how it behaves as you age will help you make more informed decisions.

When talking about skin "type," we are really talking about two different things. First, there is skin phototype or the skin color. Then we have skin classification in terms of dominant skin feature, tone, texture and signs of aging. From exfoliants and scar treatment to eye serums and sun protection, your skin care regimen is dependent on your skin phototype and dominant skin feature. This knowledge also helps you find specialists who have experience with your skin phototype. If you have a darker skin type (i.e. Asian, Hispanic, Middle Eastern, African American), having a physician or provider with experience in different skin types is especially important. It's a similar concept as going to a hair stylist with specific experience with African American hair, or a plastic surgeon with experience in the nuances of surgery for Asian eyelids. Taking these things into consideration is important, while your skin's dominant feature helps you figure out where to focus your anti-aging treatments first.

Skin Phototype and the Fitzpatrick System

Below is a basic outline of the six medically recognized skin color types based on pigmentation and sun sensitivity. This scale is known as the Fitzpatrick skin type or phototype system, developed in 1975 by Thomas

B. Fitzpatrick. [1] The system was developed after many interviews with people about skin color and how their skin was affected by sun exposure. The research revealed clear trends among different skin color types, making the Fitzpatrick system the self-assessment standard and a great tool for those wanting to better protect themselves from sun exposure.

These skin types are based on pigment and sun exposure sensitivity and do not include information about oily, dry or combination skin. I'll talk more about that later. If you have darker skin, understanding your specific needs for lasers is important, but the general concept of browning is important for all.

Skin Type 1 is highly sun-sensitive, pale with freckles and either Caucasian, possibly redhead, or albino skin. Type 1 always burns, never tans.

Skin Type 2 is commonly known as fair-skinned. Type 2s are very sun-sensitive, pale and usually burn, occasionally tanning.

Skin Type 3 is occasionally sun-sensitive but will slowly tan to a light brown. Ethnicity is typically a European mix or olive-toned Caucasian.

Skin Type 4 is minimally sun-sensitive and will tan to a darker brown. Ethnicities include Mediterranean, European, Asian, Hispanic and Native American.

Skin Type 5 is very rarely sun sensitive, tans well and rarely burns. Ethnicities include Hispanic, African American and Middle Eastern.

Skin Type 6 never burns, deeply pigmented. Ethnicities include African American, African and some darker Middle Eastern.

Let's say you're looking to invest in some laser treatment for stubborn acne pigmentation that just refuses to go away. For the sake of this example, let's also assume you have a medium skin tone (skin Phototype 3) that tans easily. The majority of testing on lasers has been done on lighter skin types. This means that while most lasers have adjustable settings depending on the skin phototype, severity and the level of penetration needed, there is still more risk with receiving certain laser treatments if you have darker skin.

This is an important factor to consider if you have darker skin: a professional who has been trained on a laser doesn't necessarily have training with a laser for your skin type. It takes a skilled and experienced practitioner to perform laser procedures on a patient with darker skin types. It is in your best interest to know your skin type and which questions to ask before receiving treatment. If the operator doesn't know to ask if you've received treatment with this laser before, or know to change levels of the skin care device based on your skin type, then that's a recipe for disaster. My point in telling you this is not to scare you, I simply want you to remember there is a person behind the procedures just as there is a person receiving treatment (you) and the lines of communication between these two people must be crystal clear. So be your own advocate and ask these questions. In fact, ask every question, it's your right. We will talk more about what questions to ask your professional later, or you can flip to the back of the book and study up now.

Although the Fitzpatrick scale only outlines six general skin color types, we know there are literally hundreds if not thousands of skin shades present in human beings. When it comes to choosing your foundation shade, this becomes a problem for pretty much everyone. Whether you wear makeup to even out your skin tone or purely for aesthetic expression, finding the perfect foundation shade is a lot like finding the perfect wedding dress. Thankfully, there are some makeup lines that are addressing this problem. Not long ago there was a limited number of foundation shades to choose from. (That's probably why I never got into makeup; I couldn't find what I needed). Today, with makeup lines producing more custom shades, we have more options to wear makeup as close to our skin phototype as possible. But with more options comes more room for error. See a makeup specialist to get matched so you don't find yourself walking around with your face a different color than your neck and chest. You should also have a winter and summer foundation shade, as you tend to tan during the summer because of longer days and more time spent outside.

CLASSIFYING DOMINANT SKIN FEATURES

The cosmetic industry has long been committed to the idea of oily, combination and dry skin as classification for cosmetics and skin care lines. There are thousands of blog posts recommending certain treatment and beauty routines based on this model. I do not agree with this model. I think it's reductive. From what I've seen, about 75 percent of my patients have combination skin, meaning parts of their face are dry and parts of their face are oily. Because of this, most of the rules separating dry skin from oily skin don't end up applying. For example, someone who has an oily T-zone, but dry cheeks should not be putting anti-oil products on their entire face. The reverse is true if someone is really dry in the perioral area and they apply moisturizer a lot they may make oily areas worse. So, if 75 percent of people really have combination skin then this dry-or-oily system is a difficult thing to choose your products based on. Additionally, your environment is changing more often than you think, which changes your skin. The seasons change, you spend more or less time outdoors, you expose yourself to extreme temperatures, you take a trip to super-humid Florida that quickly reverses when you go back to a different climate. These variables compound our problems and make it almost impossible to put one person in a "dry" box and another in an "oily" box.

If the whole goal of this model is to select a moisturizer tailored to your face. There's no harm in defining your skin in this way. However, it is not an adequate measure of treating skin issues, like acne, rosacea or pigmentation. The basic logic behind these skin care and beauty product lines is to provide a more user-friendly way to select ingredients. Dry skin products have very little alcohol, for example, while products for oily skin have more astringents. In this sense it has value when you are trying to find something to match your issue at that time. It you try something and it's too drying, then you simply experiment with the next one. People with combination skin may be able to use harsher products in their oily areas and have to be gentler on the dry areas, which the oily/dry/combination standard doesn't take into consideration.

As a dermatologist, I classify skin types a bit differently. When a patient comes into my office, I classify their skin by the dominant feature on the face that needs treatment to help the skin look better. Over the course of treatments for this dominant feature a patient's skin classification will change. I'm a great example of this. I had severe acne as an adult, so the only thing anyone saw was my acne, not wrinkles, sagging or brown spots. Once I took Accutane (the brand name for high, concentrated dose of vitamin A) the acne disappeared and now I am no longer an acne dominant skin type. I share this with you as a reminder that you absolutely have the freedom to pick a skin care line of products based on the standard dry, oil, or combination classifications and use that information to pick anti-aging products, but it does not help you treat your individual skin to affect change. To affect change, you need to use the medical or treatment classifications that we will discuss. I classify skin into seven general areas:

1. Acne Prone
2. Rosacea and redness
3. Dry and eczematous
4. Oily and sebaceous
5. Sun damaged
6. Melasma and hormonal sensitivities
7. Wrinkles

Classification 1: Acne Prone and Acne Rosacea
Acne, or appropriately called acne vulgaris in the dermatology world, is our humbling frenemy in adolescence and unfortunately affects up to 20 percent of adults. Acne is a byproduct of bacteria, abnormal cell turnover, inflammation, hormones and oil. Sometimes a specific cause like diet can be identified, but more often than not this is genetic and there is nothing the individual has done wrong. Whatever the cause, acne can play a number on our self-esteem. When a blemish forms, the inflammation, excess oil and bacteria stretch the pore and cause the red inflamed lesion you see on the surface. Deeper lesions can cause damage while under the surface your skin is pumping out anti-inflammatory mechanisms and new collagen to try to repair the tissue. This patchwork leaves noticeable scars if the lesion was deep enough (or if you picked at them!). When someone has acne, we don't see any other signs of aging, so unless we treat the acne first, other signs of aging will go untreated.

Classification 2: Rosacea Telangiectasia or Redness

Rosacea is a chronic inflammatory skin condition that affects about 1 in 20 Americans, typically those with fair skin. In my opinion there are three main types of skin rosacea: the acne type, the red type (called erythematotelangiectatic rosacea) or the sebaceous type. Of course, you can also have a combination of these types. While the exact cause of rosacea is still unknown, there are good treatments for the condition, which are based on which type of rosacea you have. Because this condition is most common on the face, I have patients coming in for treatment quite frequently. For the people with the red type of rosacea (erythematotelangiectatic) they can have flushing and growth of blood vessels on the skin. This type can be exacerbated by environmental factors like chemicals, spicy food or alcohol. Once the blood vessels become permanent, it can be treated with light that targets and destroys redness including Intense Pulse Light (IPL), pulsed dye laser or other targeted procedures.

The third type of rosacea I call sebaceous. In its mildest form, sebaceous rosacea type skin is just oilier than "normal" skin, but in time and in the more severe forms it can develop into the skin changes of phymatous rosacea, where the skin gets thick over the nose and chin or other areas on the face. W.C. Fields is a good example of this. This type when caught early is treatable with conservative measures like retinoid, peels and lasers; but once it gets to the severe form where the skin has thickened, I refer these patients to Dr. Timothy Janiga for surgical treatment of the thickened excess skin. Some people have a combination of the three types, like President Clinton. He has had redness and acne for years and has developed the thickened skin on his nose in addition as he has aged.

Despite which type of rosacea a person has, this classification can often be the most dominant feature on the face—so much so that other signs might not even be apparent until signs of rosacea are treated and under control. In addition, when prescribing or recommending anti-aging medications for rosacea patients, the dermatologist must consider factors like underlying inflammation and oil production; otherwise medication may make the dominant condition worse.

Classification 3: Dry and Eczematous

Despite the number of products out there focused on dry skin, I would say only 10 percent of the people that come into my office with dry skin as their dominant feature—and I live and work in northern Nevada, a very dry climate. People with dry skin typically also have a history of atopic dermatitis, allergies or very sensitive skin. Most of the products they have to choose are targeted toward increasing moisture. Most anti-aging products irritate them, and they are likely to also experience more prominent lines because dry skin can make wrinkles look worse. That being said, these people usually have small pores, very little acne and look quite good when they are in their 20s to 40s. As they get older it's hard to use anti-aging products because they tend to dry out the skin and these patients usually have to sacrifice anything that dried out the skin for heavy moisturization. The good news is there are topical anti-aging formulations now that do not dry out the skin and are more neutral in their effects. If you have very dry or sensitive skin your dermatologist will be able to tailor your regimen for your skin specifically.

For more information about Atopic Dermatitis, flip to the Appendix.

Classification 4: Oily or Sebaceous

Everyone needs a certain amount of natural oil to maintain healthy skin. With that said, there are people who are distinctly oily with large pores and possibly bumps from enlarged oil glands. Oily skin as a dominant feature is not that common, usually less than 10 percent in my practice. If you have this skin classification, you probably find yourself worrying about how oily or greasy your face looks throughout the day. Makeup might feel like it just slides right off, and over time you might notice the pores on your nose and cheeks are enlarged. If you have oily skin, you should use it as a gauge for which products to use. In general, people with oily skin should use oil-free sunscreens and moisturizer. They may also tolerate stronger concentrations of retinoid. It is often that the oilier you are the more drying agent you can tolerate. This allows people with oily skin to use a broader range and higher concentrations of anti-aging products. Although this type of skin may sound great to those of us with dry skin who are less tolerant to anti-aging products, when not properly cared for, this type of skin can secrete excess oil and cause thickened skin and permanently enlarge pores.

Classification 5: Sun Damage and Sunspots

Characteristically sun damaged skin can range from mild to severe and include sun spots (commonly called age spots or liver spots), collagen and elastin breakdown manifesting as texture changes, and irregularity in the pigment or even yellowing of the skin. Sunspots generally appear on parts of the body that typically get the most sun exposure: the face, neck, arms, hands, and "V" of the chest. The age spots themselves are mostly harmless for your health but are an overall indicator of your sun damage load. Be wary though. There is a type of skin cancer that can develop from a sunspot, so watch your spots for changes and have your skin checked annually. Sunspots are a common cosmetic concern treated with lasers, exfoliants, and lightening/bleaching creams. Before treating sunspots on your own, you should have a skin check with a board-certified dermatologist to confirm that these are plain sunspots.

As we have discussed already in this book, sun exposure also damages collagen and elastin. This damage is manifested by irregularities in texture. I call this cobblestoning of the skin because it looks like a cobblestone walkway if you look at it closely. This is a direct result of the damage the sun has done to the collagen and elastin in the skin and is common after many years of sun exposure. It can be treated with retinoid, laser resurfacing, and repeated chemical peels. If this is your dominant feature of your aging, this is the area you should focus.

Classification 6: Melasma and Hormonal Sensitivities

Pigmentation To understand disorders with pigmentation, we must first understand what causes the pigment in the first place. Pigment is produced by melanin in the skin, which is stimulated by ultraviolet (UV) rays and protects our skin from UV radiation. Melanin can also be stimulated by hormonal imbalance and inflammation.

A lack or overproduction of melanin can cause pigmentation inconsistencies, which vary depending on your skin type. Sun Damage is primarily responsible for pigmentation in light-skinned individuals (Types 1-3) and can often lead to hyperpigmentation or a blotchy complexion. Skin Types 5 and 6 tend to have less sun damage, but often experience genetic pigmentation problems. People of Indian descent, for example, may have darker pigment under their eyes. Melasma is a chronic skin condition that takes the form of inconsistent pigment patches on the face and body. The name comes from melas, the Greek word for black. It is most common in people with darker skin types, but also occurs frequently in lighter skin tones, though predominantly women. It is not cancerous, contagious or caused by allergies. We now know that UV rays, genetics and hormones play a part in the development of melasma.

The Difficulty With Melasma

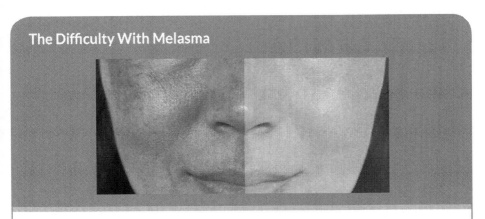

If you observe sisters, both with the same skin type and with slightly different genetic makeup, and expose them to the same amount of sun, they will get melasma differently, because they are just genetically different. Take my sister and myself for example. Our mother is Italian and the rest of our heritage is mostly Northern European, our mother does not have melasma, neither did our grandmother or great grandmother. But, both my sister and I have it. We grew up in southern Nevada before the age of sunscreen, went to camp outside every summer and had a pool in our backyard. My sister developed melasma on her upper lip mostly and a little bit on her cheeks, where mine came solely on my cheeks and my forehead in equal distribution. Both of our melasma developed in our late 20s and early 30s and we have been trying to control it since then. As I tell my patients, "melasma is the devil," it is a very difficult condition to control and women really hate it. We will likely both battle our melasma until we are fortunate enough to go through menopause, do you sense the irony?

Classification 7: Wrinkles and Sun Damage

A revered method classifying wrinkles is the Glogau Wrinkle Scale. [2] Understanding where you fall on this scale will help to determine what time of treatment you could benefit from now.

The Glogau Wrinkle Scale:

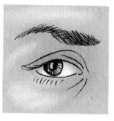 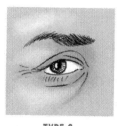 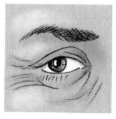 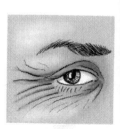

TYPE 1   TYPE 2   TYPE 3   TYPE 4

- **Type 1:** There are no wrinkles. Type 1 is classified by early photoaging, mild pigment changes; maybe some fine etchings around the eyes and virtually no age spots.
- **Type 2:** Expression lines are apparent. Type 2 is classified by early to moderate photoaging, appearance of lines only when face moves, early brown "age spots," more prominent skin pores, and early changes in skin texture.
- **Type 3:** Wrinkles visible at rest. Type 3 is classified by advanced photoaging, prominent brown pigmentation, visible brown "age spots," small blood vessels, and wrinkles present with face at rest (not when frowning or smiling).
- **Type 4:** Many wrinkles. Type 4 is classified by severe photoaging, wrinkles all over, at rest or moving, yellowish or gray skin color, skin cancers or precancerous skin changes.

For more information about special populations and conditions including those with eczema, rosacea, and acne, flip to the Appendix.

In my day-to-day practice I meet all types of people, but I have yet to meet someone over the age of thirty that does not fit into one of these dominant skin characteristics. This is why I always start here, and then move forward. While I am not opposed to the oily combination and dry skin method for choosing over the counter treatments, once you progress into the aging process you will begin to declare what your dominant features are, and we should start there. I prefer using this classification system for more effective anti-aging, prevention and maintenance treatments. While most dermatologists charge a consultation fee, it could save you a lot of money down the road that you would have spent experimenting with different over the counter treatments.

Skin: One Ever-changing Son-of-a-gun

Our skin type fluctuates depending on the season, the environment, hormones and menstrual cycle, sleep cycle, genetics and shifts in lifestyle. Environmental changes, whether caused by the seasons or other shifts, have a huge influence on your moisturization needs. Patients who come into my office regularly ask me if they are dry, oily or combination type skin. The truth is, I only see you for that small window of time, and I don't know whether you just came from the gym or you've been blasting your heater at home. I can tell you what I see today but that's only if you haven't used your oil-blotting product just prior to walking in the door. Being aware of these changes can help you choose products that are suited for your skin at that time.

Your skin changes year after year and it also changes within the year, during the different seasons, especially if you live somewhere blessed with all four seasons. The most common changes you've likely experienced is how dry and itchy your skin gets in the winter. In fact, studies show there is a higher percentage of eczema diagnoses in winter. [3] Every year as the temperature drops I get an influx of patients needing treatment for dry skin and eczema. This has a lot to do with the change in environmental humidity. Because our skin is essentially a moisture holding barrier, when the humidity levels decrease in the winter (along with increased wind), our skin increases its transepidermal evaporation—which is just a fancy term for moisture leaving the skin. There's a natural decrease in environmental humidity coupled with more fireside time and cranking up the heaters in our homes. Our car heaters and warm office spaces not only encourage dry skin, these environments basically invite dry skin in for a cup of coffee. Though humid climates do help most people, I personally recommend using thicker moisturizer in the winter and more often. Try to use less drying products, like reducing the retinoid from twice a week to once a week. Increasing exfoliation with an alpha hydroxy acid during winter months can also help dry skin by bringing in moisture and improving cell turnover. Humidity levels decrease in the winter (along with increased wind), our skin increases its transepidermal evaporation—which is just a fancy term for moisture leaving the skin. There's a natural decrease in environmental humidity coupled with more fireside time and cranking up the heaters in our homes. Our car heaters and warm office spaces not only encourage dry skin, these environments basically invite dry skin in for a cup of coffee. Though humid climates do help most people, I personally recommend using thicker moisturizer in the winter and more often. Try to use less drying products, like reducing the retinoid from twice a week to once a week. Increasing exfoliation with an alpha hydroxy acid during winter months can also help dry skin by bringing in moisture and improving cell turnover. If you're looking for all the help you can get, adding a moisturizing mask once a week can also help replenish some moisture and keep that skin barrier strong.

Aging & Beauty Industry and Culture

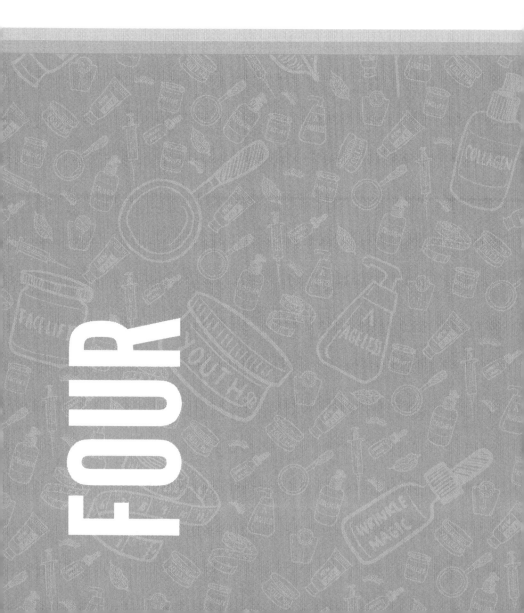

FOUR

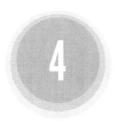

AGING & BEAUTY INDUSTRY AND CULTURE

The average American woman applies a minimum of 16 cosmetic products on her face every day and spends roughly $250 per month on beauty and skin care products. High fashion publications churn out monthly spreads of beauty and anti-aging tips, highlighting the latest products used by the famous, the wealthy and the "it" girls of the moment to keep up with the standard. [1] Our selection of safe and effective anti-aging methods is only growing, as the business of anti-aging stands at $118 billion and is projected to become a $1 trillion market by 2025. [2]

In the United States—and much of Western culture in general—the aging woman has not been featured in these ads and brochures. Western culture has gone to great lengths to remain looking young, and the industry goes to great lengths to keep up with (and cultivate) the demand. In my line of work, I am thankful to have access to top-of-the-line anti-aging technologies and products to have the knowledge to know what is best and to use them. My face and my look could be considered an advertisement for my work—just like you wouldn't want to get a game changing hair cut from a stylist who looks unkempt, patients would be a bit confused if I didn't have personal experience with fillers, lasers, topicals and neuromodulators.

AMERICAN CULTURAL STANDARD AND DEMAND

The American Cultural Standard of beauty updates every so often, historically speaking about every decade. Think of the evolution of the ideal eyebrow, for instance. There were the ultra-thin eyebrows of the Roaring Twenties; the thick, well-defined eyebrows of the '50s pin-up era; the bushy brow of the '80s made famous by Brooke Shields; the pencil-thin eyebrows of the '90s (think Courtney Cox) and now we have moved the pendulum back again to thicker eyebrows. These are trends, and while we all can't help but keep up with the times, all that truly matters is that you feel comfortable, confident and beautiful in your own skin. Ask yourself: what does beauty mean to you? Do you have a sense of vitality? What makes you feel beautiful? What gives you confidence? Knowing where you stand with these questions can help you have a better understanding of your cosmetic desires and empower you to be your best advocate.

It is natural to compare how we look to others to gauge where we sit on the beauty and aging spectrum. But that comparison can easily be skewed, based on our environment (there's that learned perception of beauty again!). While comparing ourselves to others can be a bit of a slippery slope, there is some science behind why we feel the need to do this in the first place. Research shows women befriend other women who are similar in attractiveness. This is another one of those evolutionary leftovers, think about finding a mate in the caveman days and this makes sense. In the study researchers took photos of 46 different female friends and had both subjects and outside judges rate the relative attractiveness of the friends. The women were then tasked with rating their friendships, expressing their level of agreement with questions like, "Is it more difficult for me to meet men when my friend is around?" While more research is needed in this area, the current study suggests women who have friends with similar attractiveness are less competitive with one another.

Friends also influence things like body image. For example, "skinny" is a pretty subjective term, but we all use it. It's a standard term in American culture. The strong influence of the Western culture to be "skinny" [1] is the backbone of fat reduction procedures; but the way we each perceive skinny, and what that means for you, is largely dependent on what our inner circle perceives as skinny. [3] The same goes with aging. No one wants to feel like the oldest-looking one in the group. These are all topics that come up when considering cosmetic procedures.

Several of my patients have come into my office wanting a lift here or some filler there because they feel they look older than their counterparts. Some even choose to keep these procedures secret. Whether it's a personal privacy thing or they're afraid to be called out, I do think this should change. The more open we are about these procedures, the more realistic our expectations as a group can be. Wanting to put our best face forward is inherently human and nothing to be ashamed of. Ironically, these comparisons to our age counterparts (think Andie MacDowell and that TV commercial for anti-aging products) as well as our evolutionary desire to look like our friends are a couple of the powerful tactics brands can use to convince us we need their products.

A MASERATI WITHOUT AN ENGINE

I went to San Francisco a few months ago with my sister-in-law and I experienced firsthand the masterful persuasion of professionals in the anti-aging and beauty industry. This was an extraordinarily eye-opening sales experience that clarified the imposing nature of beauty brands on our everyday lives.

We were in the shopping district looking for shoes one moment and the next we found ourselves lured into a high-end skin care boutique. I am not sure how I even ended up in there, I think he complimented us on how pretty we looked, and voila, we were inside. The store opened up into this 3,000-square-foot showroom filled with women—some with hand mirrors in front of them, others standing in line at demo stations. The young doorman/model asked what I did for a living in an Eastern European accent. I said I was a mom. I wasn't lying, but I didn't want our experience tainted by their knowledge of my professional background. I immediately thought that I wanted the experience that my patients would have if they were in this store. I was curious, so I looked over at my sister-in-law and whispered, "Don't tell them I'm a dermatologist. Let's just have some fun." After a quick glance at my face and a few strategic complements about my age, the associate sat us down at an area with the skin care line he thought was best for us. He brought us some wine "so the tired moms could spend some time on themselves for once." Oh he was good! Looking around while he got our wine, the other groups of women were accompanied by different young men with accents (by now I was sure everyone had to have an accent to work there). There was one token older woman who assisted women near the makeup section, and she also had an accent. *Oh good,* I thought, *they at least have someone age-matched to relate to* (think Andie MacDowell again). Smart.

In the name of research (and intrigue), I allowed the salesman to apply products to one side of my face and see what it was like. The vaguely European man raved about its miraculous ability to remove dead skin cells, so I figured I'd give it a go. This cleanser beads up as you rub it on your face, and the beads are supposedly all your dead skin sloughing off your face. They tell me to use it once a week, so I bought the cleanser. He then applied an eye serum and cream to only one side of my face. He did the opposite side on my sister-in-law. How curious? Not really! In the industry it is common practice to look at the subject's face and apply creams to the better side, so when you look in the mirror you see that the applied side is "better." We are all asymmetric. We usually have sun damage on one side more than the other, and usually driving side is worse. He used this technique on us. I usually drive so my left side is worse. My sister-in-law is more often the passenger so her right side was the worse side. In addition, simply adding hydration to our skin did make us look better in that area, it changes the way light reflects off the skin, making it look smoother and less crepe-like.

Being the scientist at heart that I am, I went home and washed my face with the aforementioned cleanser and saw the skin ball up on my face just like it did during the demo with the handsome guy. I washed my faced a second time and the same amount of "skin" balled up all over my face before I rinsed it off again. So, I did this 45 times, which I don't recommend, but I was on a mission. The same amount of "skin" balled up each of the 45 times. After the 45th time, it's not really dead skin exfoliating anymore. Then again, it was a nice enough cleanser, I did like it, and there were some good ingredients in it. But it wasn't just that. It was the full experience that came with the cleanser. It was the way the on-site esthetician/sales associate demonstrated products on my face, taking special care to apply products to the less sun-damaged side to reveal a more dramatic before-and-after effect. I was being told I looked 15 years younger now than my driver's license photo when I paid (Side-note: my driver's license was only 2 months old. He did not look that closely at the date).

I was sitting in the chair waiting for the complimentary facial I received as part of my purchase and expressed I did not receive regular facials. That was like the kiss of death there, and they spent the entirety of my facial trying to convince me I might spontaneously combust into an old lady because of my lack of facials. I happen to know that this is not true, so it did not bother me; but would it have bothered one of my patients? Would she have been guilted into purchasing a package of facials or say, "no thank you," and still feel that she is not taking good care of herself? In my office I try hard to give people the best advice based on their situation and not guilt people into purchases or treatments. None of these things are life or death (and definitely no risk of spontaneous combustion). There are many limitations on what we are able to do for ourselves, including time, money and access to babysitters for our children. We are doing what we can and deserve no guilt about it.

As I was checking out after my facial, I had not purchased the full series of products he had used on me during the facial. He tried one last time to get me to purchase more by giving me a steep discount because "he liked me so much." I said, "No thank you," and that I wanted to try what I had first. If I liked it, I would come back for the others. He let me know that I had a "Maserati without the engine" and my products and regiment were not complete. I laughed a little at the terminology. It was really catchy; but again, I thought of my patients and what they might do in this situation.

The store I went to was just one of four other similar boutiques on that street. This type of experiential marketing is very much the new norm and people like it. They get personal service, wine and a great looking young guy giving them compliments for an hour. We certainly had a great time. It was fun to be swept away into a different world and "shown the ropes." The associates make it fun and it was great to be pampered. As the dermatologist, once the pampering and wine was over, it came to me that this was a complete microcosm of everything we are talking about in this book. By no means am I saying you should avoid these places all together. It was fun for us. I only ask you to consider the messenger's motives.

This type of marketing happens to most of us now in smaller doses, in similar but slightly different forms. It occurs in infomercials, makeup counters and kiosks at the mall. I remember a long-time patient of mine came in and asked me about getting filler instead of BOTOX®. She saw in a magazine that Christie Brinkley prefers this method because it looks more natural. I told her that, for the treatment she wanted, the filler was not really indicated for that area would be more expensive and has higher risks. She got that angry face. "I fell for it! I can't believe I fell for it!" This patient is an incredibly smart professional woman, and she was susceptible to the celebrity endorsement disguised in an editorial. She thanked me for the honest and safer treatment.

My patients have a long-term relationship with me for many years, and it is my priority to help patients get the products and treatments they need when they need it, no sooner and no later. You will hear me say, "Your face is my face!" which is why I chose the products I sell in my office because they are effective, not because I get a commission on them. Like any of my reputable colleagues, I encourage my patients to use what works for them. They have time to discuss best options with me and then come back anytime in the next 20 years to get it. Oftentimes the products that work for them are not the products that I offer, whether it's a decision of preference or cost. We can always add products later if a dominant feature of aging becomes more prominent.

Navigating the Skin Care Aisle
There are hundreds of brands out there. Some are endorsed by celebrities with beautiful skin, most with pretty models on the display; and others are endorsed by dermatologists to emphasize the medical or cosmetic integrity. But, there is no need to have them all in your beauty cabinet. So, how do you choose? There are a handful of ingredients that have been scientifically shown to aid in the protection, maintenance and improvement of your skin as you age, and the goal is to have proper concentrations of these in your beauty regimen based on your age, skin type and cosmetic goals.

Some of these essentials (i.e. antioxidants and retinoid) are mass marketed as a spotlight ingredient in brand-name creams. However, because the Federal Drug Administration (FDA) does not regulate cosmeceutical products, the concentration levels are not always clear for cosmeceuticals.

In contrast, Retin-A is an FDA-approved prescription and comes in concentrations of 0.025 percent, 0.05 percent and 0.1 percent. Not unlike all industries, strategic marketing language can sometimes be misleading. For these reasons it is important to pay attention to why you buy certain products. Depending on the amount of change or improvement you hope to achieve with any given product or procedure, it's best to consult your dermatologist. This is especially true if you are looking for a certain ingredient to help with a specific aging issue. A physician-dispensed or prescription-strength product tailored to your specific needs will almost always give you better results than a mass-marketed product.

Cosmeceuticals are strictly meant for *cosmetic* use. They do not have any pharmaceutical regulations to follow. Think about what the TV commercial would be like for these cosmeceuticals if they had to do what prescription medications did—that fast-talking guy at the end rushing through side effects and results. Because anti-aging products are mass-marketed, the claims can be borderline grandiose. However, highly targeted, fine-tuned marketing of cosmetics is fair game. Therefore, it is up to the consumer to make educated decisions by knowing fact from fiction (and all the gray area in between). But with so many new, improved and glamorous options out there, weeding through the clutter can be easier said than done.

WHERE SHOULD I START?

When I sit with a new patient for a consultation, I hand them a mirror and say, "Point to what bothers you." That's where we start, because we want to address the dominant feature of aging, or what bothers *you*—not what a friend may have received, or a magazine may have featured. Physical signs of aging can make us eager to try new, cutting edge treatments, especially if it comes highly recommended by a friend. Though, committing to treatments prior to consultation can distract us from the specific dominant features that make us feel older in the first place. Knowing the specifics of what bothers you can help guide your ideal treatment plan.

While no one person will have the same introduction into cosmetic treatment, I generally recommend starting with preventive measures like sunscreen and antioxidants before procedures. Think of it like building a house. If you don't start with a solid foundation, then even the sturdiest house will end up with cracks. The exception, of course, is if you're dealing with reconstructive needs or any other urgent medical situation.

If you are protecting your skin, and you're finding it might be time for the next level of treatment, your dermatologist can help guide you to the next step that is best for you. I often have patients who see me because they think they need a surgical procedure when really that is too aggressive of an option for them at that time. Other times I have patients who have successfully avoided surgery with noninvasive procedures for years but are now at a stage where surgery is the next necessary step (based on their goals). Noninvasive procedures are cheaper than surgery, but that doesn't always mean they are the best option for you and what you're trying to accomplish. On that same note, just because you have the budget for a full facelift, neck lift and fat grafting, doesn't mean you need that right now.

If a surgical procedure is in the cards, taking steps in prevention and maintenance will help you protect your investment in these procedures. For example, if you are planning on having a facelift, you will need to stop smoking for safety. During the preparation process for a facelift in our office, I will often meet with the patient and start a skin care regimen or tweak the current one to best protect the investment they have made in the facelift. Additionally, I may recommend a laser resurfacing treatment if they have some sun damage that could benefit from that. Giving your skin plenty of antioxidants, stimulating cell turnover with retinoid and growth factors, and protecting your skin from sun damage with a broad-spectrum SPF will strengthen your skin and decrease the repair needed in the future.

The noninvasive treatment industry is advancing more quickly than ever. Laser and injection treatments can be performed on your lunch break. Fat reduction procedures are done in an afternoon. While in the past your options were either surgery or a chemical peel and nothing in between, now there are many options, and you can choose where and when you start. As technologies continually upgrade to meet the no downtime, minimal-risk requests of our patients, the results available from these less invasive procedures continue to improve. Though it will be quite a long time, if ever, that noninvasive will eclipse surgery when it comes to results, they are getting better all the time and allow small improvements to be done before larger procedures become a patient's best option. An example of an area that can be treated with noninvasive options or surgery is the fat pad below the chin. This area can be treated with an injectable product such as deoxycholic acid (i.e. Kybella®), a fat sculpting device (i.e. CoolSculpting®), or liposuction and a neck lift. The first two will not help the extra skin around the fat pad as much as the surgical option will. There is sort of a point of no return, a checkpoint for qualifying for noninvasive treatments. When you really need a neck lift to reach the results you're trying to achieve, no amount of Kybella® or CoolSculpting® is going to get you there.

The worlds of dermatology and plastic surgery often overlap, and it's beneficial for practitioners in both fields to have connections in the other. In my practice, I have the option of referring patients to my husband, Dr. Timothy Janiga, a board-certified plastic surgeon, if indeed plastic surgery is the best option. if someone comes to me for a noninvasive procedure that I know will not achieve the results they are requesting, I can refer them to my husband. Talk with your practitioner to decide the best option for your goals, even if the best option is something they do not offer and you need to be referred to another specialist. Go with the treatment that is most likely to get you to the results you're trying to achieve. It's about what's best for you, the one making the investment. However, generally speaking, most people that I talk with are interested in making changes and improvements on the area of their bodies that gets the most attention—the face.

PUT YOUR MONEY WHERE YOUR FACE IS:

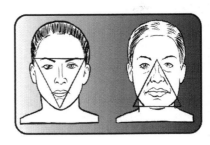

Special Considerations for Your Face, Neck and Chest

Prioritizing one procedure over another can be difficult since most people are (understandably) unsure where to start. If you find yourself torn between doing a body procedure or a facial procedure, I recommend choosing the face since it's the first feature people see. We use the face to read and interact with others. It is also one of the most exposed areas along with the neck, chest and hands. This exposure to elements leads to earlier signs of aging than less exposed areas like abdomen, arms and legs. When we determine someone's age, we create our first impression of a person by looking at the upper third of the face, which includes the eyes and brow line, as well as the **triangle of youth**: the cheeks, nose and upper lip (We'll expand on these in this chapter). Then our eyes venture down to the lower half of the face, neck and chest. If you have a few different things that need to be treated on the face, such as brown spots, volume loss and wrinkles, always treat your dominant aging feature first. This will give you the most result first. Here we will take a look at special considerations for the face, neck and chest. This includes treatments and procedures for eyelashes, eyebrows, eyelids, lips, neck and chest.

The Window to Your Age: The Eyes

As the most captivating and emotive feature of the face, the eyes speak our truths before anything else, and that includes our age. The eyes are usually the first feature we see in one another. Aging skin around the eyes tends to make us look more tired than we really are. This is because of the delicate, significantly thinner skin framing the eyes. The skin keeps getting thinner as we age, revealing signs of fine lines, age and spots while making the tissues more prone to environmental damage. While taking care of yourself will certainly help defend your body against early signs of aging, collagen eventually breaks down and those fine lines and wrinkles need a little extra help. In time, we acquire skin laxity as well, which leads to a host of issues, including dark circles, bags, puffiness, fine lines and wrinkles. Drooping of the skin, in its most severe form, can cause vision problems and can lead to the feeling that you look tired all the time.

The eye is as intricate as it is sensitive, and so you might find the way your eyes age is different than your friends. The main aging issues people experience are dark circles, bags and crow's feet.

Dark Circles and Pigmentation

Dark circles are one of the most common reasons that patients come see me. Dark circles are caused by a number of factors that I categorize as superficial, deep or physiologic. Superficial causes of dark circles include pigmentation, skin thinning and superficial blood vessels in the skin. Thinning skin under the eyes is a common issue. The thin skin becomes almost transparent and gives a hollow, bluish discoloration. The eyelid skin is the most sensitive skin on the body and does not tolerate a lot of products that other skin on the face can. A dedicated eye cream is always the best option.

Be Careful, Sensitive Skin Types!

A few years back I was at a dermatology conference, and it wasn't until the first night that I realized I had forgotten my face wash at home. My friend let me borrow hers, but when I woke up the next morning my eyes were swollen shut. The irony was thick as I walked around the dermatology conference with swollen eyelids for 2 days. Thankfully the setting worked in my favor too, and I was able to grab some samples from various booths to treat myself. At any rate, my experience underlines how sensitive the eyelid skin can be in some people, including me.

Pigmentation underneath the eyes is either acquired over time through lack of sleep, dehydration and gradual aging, or caused by genetics based on your heritage (We will get to that in a minute). Despite the cause, pigmentation is difficult to treat. For acquired pigmentation, gentle use of lightening creams, sunscreen and antioxidants can help. Again, specific eye creams are usually the best for this area tailored to you. Laser can be used to treat superficial blood vessels, but make sure you are with a qualified provider, since laser around the eyes requires a few extra preparation steps. If you are close to the eye you may need to wear eye shields inside your lids (like a contact lens) to treat these more difficult vessels.

Deep causes of dark circles include volume loss and visibility of deeper veins beneath the skin. Volume loss can be treated with specialized fillers that are designated for this sensitive area. To reduce the margin for error as much as possible, only a very experienced provider should treat this area with filler. This is not an FDA-approved indication for the fillers like Juvéderm® and Restylane®, but an experienced provider can go through this with you. The deeper veins are more difficult to treat. They can be covered with makeup or treated by a vein specialist with injections. Again, the eye area is very specific and sensitive, so only an experienced vein specialist should do this.

Physiologic causes of dark circles include sinus issues, allergies and genetic pigmentation. Sinus issues and allergies cause fluid in the sinus cavity under the eyelid skin and can contribute to the circles that you see in the mirror. A board-certified ear, nose and throat physician or your primary care doctor is best equipped to help you with these problems. They may prescribe a nasal spray and/or antihistamine. In more extreme cases of allergies and sinus problems, surgical intervention is required, but I would not recommend sinus surgery solely to improve under-eye darkness or bags.

Genetic pigmentation under the eye is the other type of physiologic pigmentation. This is common in people with darker skin, specifically people of Hispanic or Indian descent. I find this type of pigmentation the most difficult for patients. They will usually say that they have had darkness under the eye since they were kids, but it continues to worsen as they get older. This type of pigmentation takes a combination approach of lightening creams, sunscreen, antioxidants, lasers and chemical peels. We can usually achieve a lighter skin tone in these areas, but the pigmentation usually does not go away completely.

There are hundreds of eye creams intended to treat pigmentation and dark circles, but this is a complex problem and may need more than one treatment to improve. It would be best to see your dermatologist for an evaluation of the type of pigment you have and get a treatment plan tailored to your specific type of under-eye circles.

Bags and Puffy Eyes
Bags under the eyes can be swelling, hereditary or because of aging. First let's discuss the swelling part. After having a sodium-packed meal, like sushi and soy sauce, I wake up the next morning with puffiness under my eyes. I call this "sushi eyes." This type of swelling is only temporary and may come with illness, high sodium-content food or even too much alcohol. This type of swelling under the eyes goes away within a day or so and is not a cause for concern, but you may avoid the situations that cause it if you would like to avoid it. Personally, I love soy sauce and

sushi enough to endure this transient swelling, but to each their own. The other reason for the appearance of bags under the eyes is actually not a bag. It is a sort of illusion caused by volume loss in the tear trough area. This causes a hollowing that looks like a half circle under the eye. This volume loss is treated with a small amount of volume in the form of filler or fat to decrease the contrast between the cheek and the indentation of the trough. Another cause of bags under the eyes is the weakening of the orbital septum, or the part of the eyes that holds fat in the under-eye area. This can be hereditary or acquired with aging. This is a common problem for the women in my family. I can remember my great-grandmother, grandmother and mother with this, and even myself as young as 30 with the early signs. As the orbital septum weakens, the fat is free to push outward against the skin, making it look like a protuberant fat pad. This can be treated in its early stages with filler to improve the contour, which is what I currently have. As it progresses, this fat pad usually requires surgical intervention to reposition that fat pad and tighten up the structures around it.

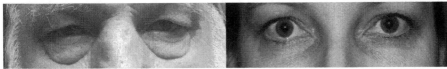

FAT HERNIATION   TEAR TROUGH

Crow's Feet

Crow's feet are a common initial sign of aging around the eyes. Crow's feet are caused by a combination of things, such as thinning skin, loss of collagen and elastin, accumulation of free radicals in the skin from pollution/environmental factors and years of smiling and squinting. I categorize crow's feet as either dynamic or static. Dynamic lines are the type of lines that only form when you are moving and completely go away when you are in a resting position. These are the earliest phase of crow's feet. After you have etched those dynamic lines for years, they can become static facial lines. Static lines begin to etch in the skin and are present with or without facial expression. Some patients etch their crow's feet as early as in their 20s, but others do not have this problem until well into their 40s. I have sent patients away and told them to come back in 5 years when they start to "etch" those lines. But, there are some people who subscribe to the concept of prevention, and I am happy to treat those people.

The most cost-effective way to prevent crow's feet is to use your expressive muscles less. That includes diminishing squinting and smiling. But where's the fun in that? There are plenty of procedures that can help repair crow's feet, so you don't have to stop smiling. Using tried and true, scientifically-backed ingredients will be your first line of defense against crow's feet (Retinoids and antioxidants, we're looking at you!). Next, in-office procedures like lasers and injectables can prevent them from getting deeper. If you plan on tackling crow's feet with a "crow's feet eye cream" make sure it includes a collagen stimulator like peptides, retinoid in low concentrations and/or growth factors. These creams will not prevent new lines from forming. For that you will need botulinum toxin A injections, commonly known BOTOX® or Dysport® injections. Crow's feet can also be softened with resurfacing procedures including radiofrequency and laser resurfacing. I typically recommend a combination of injections, resurfacing and topical creams for long-term improvement and maintenance.

If you want to make significant strides in creating a youthful impression, treat the skin around the eyes first. Your dermatologist can treat the skin laxity with specific lasers and can use filler to reshape the boney changes and give back some of that volume that has been lost over time.

Brown Spots
Brown spots (also known as age spots, sun spots or liver spots) typically show on a spectrum of light brown to grey or black. Brown spots are a sign of sun damage or too much time in the tanning bed. Brown spots typically show up in the areas of the skin most often exposed to the sun: the face, neck, chest, hands, shoulders and forearms. Those most at risk of getting brown spots have light skin, and they will begin to form in people around 40 years old, depending on how well that person protects their skin from sun damage. While brown spots are a cosmetic issue for many, they are not dangerous. You can treat brown spots with bleaching creams, intense pulse light therapy, laser therapy, chemical peels and retinoids.

Blood Vessels
Blood vessels are those small, red web-like lines that appear beneath skin, typically on the face or on the legs. Blood vessels occur with chronic sun exposure and other harsh environmental stressors, pregnancy or skin conditions like erythematotelangiectatic rosacea. While they are not

harmful, they are another one of those pesky signs of aging we'd rather do without. Blood vessels can be minimized with sunscreen and treated with intense pulse light therapy, laser therapy and redness-reducing topicals.

EYELASH GROWTH

Long, luscious eyelashes are among the top features synonymous with femininity and youth, so of course it is a bit concerning when they begin to thin. Eyelash thinning, shortening and lightening naturally occur as we age. Eyelash damage and breakage can occur from overuse of eyelash curlers and certain waterproof mascaras. Fortunately, there are several treatments to replenish your lashes. For example, there are FDA-approved, daily-use liquid products that you brush on your lash line. A 10-week supply of prescription eyelash growth product will cost you around $150, and lash growth is noticeable after 8-12 weeks. This product must be purchased in a doctor's office or at a pharmacy, as this is a prescription-only medication that you cannot get over the counter. This product was actually created after an interesting discovery from patients using an anti-glaucoma drug formula. Patients who used this drug to treat their glaucoma were growing envy-worthy eyelashes, and so this new lash-growing liquid (commonly known by the brand name, LATISSE®) was discovered. Prescriptions products like LATISSE® will lengthen and thicken the lashes as well as make them darker so they are easier to see.

If topicals on your lashes isn't your thing, you can also receive eyelash extensions. Unlike those clunky, costumey false lashes you can buy at the drugstore, eyelash extensions use a specific adhesive that allows for the aesthetician to attach an extension to individual lashes. Eyelash extensions last for 6-8 weeks, which is great if you simply want to experiment with them. If you plan on making these a standard part of your beauty routine, remember you're signing up for consistent upkeep. Some people have no problem with this and are in love with extensions, but for a busy person like me I'd rather stick to mascara and my Latisse that I can do at home.

For something a little more permanent, new advancements in technology have made eyelash transplants possible as well. This procedure is similar to eyebrow transplants and therefore should be done by a qualified physician.

The eyelashes lay at specific angles that, if applied improperly, could lead to bothersome or unruly lashes. This person is also working closely around your sensitive eyes, so do your research before jumping into the chair. This is done by a doctor and requires a surgical procedure. Like eyebrow transplants, your new hair will need to be trimmed because the hair came from an area on your head that grows longer strands.

Most over-the-counter options are eyelash enhancers with conditioners or thickeners, which work to improve the way your current eyelashes look and feel. They don't necessarily grow new lashes, but for some people this is enough or even a great place to start. Remember that eyelashes are like other hair but more fragile, so treat them with care as you cleanse your face and apply makeup. Wash makeup off with a quality eye makeup remover and never scrub it off or pick. This can cause damage to the already fragile eyelash. Take care and only use products that are made for the eyes in this area. Your sight is a precious thing, after all.

EYELID SERUMS AND RESURFACING

Eyelid Serums and Creams
Our delicate eyelids benefit from eye-specific serums that help thicken the skin around the area and reduce that crepey texture. Serums tend to be more liquidy than creams but choosing between the two is really a personal preference thing. I prefer creams as I have very dry skin and they are more moisturizing. Anti-aging eyelid creams or serums can contain a retinol, antioxidants, peptides, caffeine, hydroxy acids, moisturizers, hyaluronic acid or, more recently, ceramides. When looking at the ingredients, remember that they will do similar things for the skin around the eyes that they do for the face, but eye products are formulated to be gentler. Eye creams and serums usually have less of the irritating ingredients like retinol and hydroxy acids. I recommend using a reputable line for eye creams and trying a small area on one eye first for a few days prior to putting it all over upper and lower lids to make sure you are not sensitive to it.

Periocular Laser Resurfacing
Better known as eyelid resurfacing, this procedure improves the overall texture and complexion of the skin and tissue around the eyes. This

procedure is a safe and common procedure for those who many not need or are not yet ready for eyelid surgery, especially if you have crow's feet, moderate lines, mild tissue laxity, or age spots and pigmentation. Resurfacing around the eyes is a more advanced technique and should be performed with special precautions and safety equipment.

EYEBROWS

When we talk about eyebrows we're really talking about two features: the eyebrow hairs and the brow bone itself. Eyebrows are funny, they can give your age away, but they can also be manipulated to make you look younger. With proper care, eyebrows can become one of the key features that keep you looking younger longer. In fact, for many people, having their eyebrows done can take a few years off of their look. Maintenance of your eyebrows sits on a spectrum, from tweezing and waxing to dying to more permanent treatments like microblading and eyebrow transplants followed by surgical brow lift procedures.

Microblading
This service is great for anyone who wants his or her brows reshaped, reconstructed or thickened. Professionals numb the area with a topical anesthetic and then hash the skin with a microblading pen to recreate the look of individual hairs, and then pigment is placed in the skin in the new made hair areas. Because it requires a steady hand and great attention to detail it can take about 2 hours the first time. Practitioners have a specific certification to be qualified to perform this procedure. Patients are advised to keep the brows moist and avoid all exfoliating products until the area has healed. I get mine done and I definitely prefer this procedure to tattooing, although it's of course a personal choice. The first time I had it done, I barely felt a thing. The second time I did it without the prescription-strength anesthetic and it hurt more; therefore, I do recommend finding a practitioner affiliated with a physician office, so you can get a prescription-strength topical anesthetic. This process has brought my eyebrows and the eyebrows of many of my patients back to a more youthful appearance

Eyebrow Tattooing

Eyebrow tattooing is the more permanent predecessor to microblading, but it is still used often. This procedure is performed by a qualified makeup tattoo professional and can be done by hand or with a machine. There are several different eyebrow styles a professional can give you, depending on your preference. If you're interested in having your eyebrows tattooed but have never undergone a procedure like this, I would recommend trying microblading first, as it lasts a maximum of 18 months.

Eyebrow Transplants

Like eyelash transplants, eyebrow transplants are a surgical procedure performed by a qualified physician. In addition to microblading and makeup, brow transplants can be used to give youth to the eyebrows. This is an in-office procedure with potential for bruising and swelling afterward, but minimal risk. Take care to see an experienced eyebrow transplant doctor, as the design of the eyebrow and placement of the hairs is a technical and permanent procedure.

Shaping and Makeup

Strong, healthy eyebrows are synonymous with youth, and thinning eyebrows are one of the first things to give your age away. Thanks to the world's wax and wane affinity for thick, bold eyebrows or clean, thin and polished brows, eyebrow pencils can be found virtually anywhere. Additionally, the overwhelming influx of how-to eyebrow tutorials could keep you busy for years. However, tutorials can be tricky as they are created to benefit thousands of people, and you are one in a million.

Your level of comfort with eyebrow makeup will help determine your personal regimen for them. If you already know what works for you in the eye makeup department, good for you! I know some women who can draw on a pair of eyebrows in the back of a taxi on a winding road. I also know some women who couldn't tell you the difference between eyeliner and an eyebrow pencil.

If you've never had your eyebrows shaped, I highly recommend treating it the same way you treat your seasonal haircut and color. Get it done by a professional. Eyebrows have a way of making or breaking your look, so trusting a professional to get the correct shape is well worth the money.

He or she can help you identify what works for your unique look, how that look should update as you age, and how to avoid trends that could end up aging you. If your eyebrows are more on the bushy side, spending $30 to have them shaped can dramatically lift your eyes (and save you a few thousand dollars). The idea is to clear area between your brows and your eyelids. It's all in the optics.

Makeup As We Age

Some makeup trends simply don't look good on older women. There, I said it (but I wasn't the first!). In fact, as I entered my 40s I had to learn a few lessons myself. Sure, I want to shimmer like the best of them, but after meeting with a makeup professional I know that it is not appropriate for me to have shiny dewy cheeks. Just as my patients trust my recommendations, I trust my makeup professional with their expertise. She tells me what new colors are available and gives me makeup that works for my age. One of the main takeaways I learned from her was the concept of color and texture and how those options change (and in some cases, narrow) as you get older. For example, she took away my shimmer, but that's OK because apparently shimmer looks stupid on a 45-year-old woman. I would have never known. Caked makeup around the eyes is another great example, since it settles in our fine lines and accentuates them. Stick with a light foundation and apply with a brush. The same goes for matte lipstick. Gloss looks better on aging lips, as it does not run into our lip lines.

Botox for the Brow

While aging eyes make you look tired, drooping brow lines can have you looking chronically exhausted. A popular, noninvasive treatment for drooping brows is neuromodulator procedures. This gives a subtle lift to the brows and lasts for about 3 months. Despite the modest lift, since BOTOX® (and its competition, Dysport®) has become popularized many people prefer to go with this minimally invasive option first. According to the 2017 American Society of Plastic Surgeons (ASPS) Annual

Procedural Statistics, neuromodulators are the top minimally invasive procedure performed in the U.S.

THE TRIANGLE OF YOUTH

Below the eyes we have what we call the triangle of youth: an inverted triangle with the base at the high cheekbones to the point of the triangle at the defined jawbone. This shape is a major subconscious indicator of someone's physical age. With age we lose volume and lift, and the triangle naturally becomes more of an oblong shape. Maintaining the inverted triangle shape can be achieved with a combination of filler, tightening procedures and Botox.

Lips

Lips have a uniquely sensual and romantic impression, particularly when they're young, soft and full of collagen. For women specifically, the lips tend to be the most sexually attractive feature on the face. For this reason, it's no surprise that filler and BOTOX® for lip enhancement and reshaping are some of the more commonly requested noninvasive facial procedures I perform. The lips are composed of six areas: the oral commissures, the philtrum columns, cupid's bow, the lower lips or "pillows," the vermilion-cutaneous junction and the nasolabial creases. There are plenty of makeup options to reshape the lips, but if you're not into lip liners, you might consider lip-plumping cosmetics. Granted, these cosmetics won't make drastic changes, but they do help manipulate the optics so your lips appear fuller and have a more defined Cupid's bow. Lip plumping glosses and balms typically have an irritant in them that causes redness and swelling. Keep this in mind if you're allergy prone. Some of these tingling sensations are caused by menthol. As far as those "collagen-boosting" lip plumpers go, the key ingredient is alpha-hydroxy acids, which may help increase collagen slightly over time.

Hyaluronic acid filler in the lips has become extremely popular, too. Younger women are looking for more voluptuous pouts, while older women are simply looking to replenish the volume lost with age.

Upper lip lines (sometimes called smoker's lines or lipstick lines) begin to form in the same way that crow's feet begin, with expression lines, but also from smoking and other environmental stressors. Lip lines do form for similar reasons; though, the breakdown of collagen and elastin in the area are from aging. Lip lines can be prevented and treated in the same ways that other fine lines and wrinkles can be.

For fine lines around the lips, we have perioral laser resurfacing or Radiofrequency, which are specifically designed to improve the appearance of fine lines and wrinkles caused by sun damage and movement around the mouth. These types of treatments go deeper than microdermabrasion and chemical peels and can be adjusted in intensity depending on the level of correction needed. Recovery times vary about 2-7 days.

The Jawline

As we lose volume in the cheeks, the skin begins to loosen and sag, which softens the prominence of the jawline. This is referred to as jowls, or the sagging skin beneath the jawline. The most effective noninvasive methods for reducing jowls are to keep up with fillers to lift the face like Restylane® Lyft and JUVÉDERM VOLUMA® and tightening procedures such as Contoura Forma Plus. For minimally invasive tightening of the jowls there is FaceTite™. Once you have received these treatments, you would be ready to discuss surgery with your plastic surgeon.

NECK AND CHEST

The neck and chest are often neglected, even though this area typically gets the same amount of sun exposure as the face. In dermatology, the general rule of caring for the neck and chest is to treat the area considered "the face" starting from the nipple line up to the hairline, and to treat the area considered "the body" as if it starts from the jawline down to your toes. This way, your neck and chest get the care and benefits from both areas.

Neck creams have only recently become popular, so I'm seeing more people in their 40s and older are eager to try a product that helps add firmness to an aging, sagging neck. Though with so many neck products available over the counter, you have to wonder how many of them actually work. Using the same logic that there is no "facelift in a jar." You will be hard pressed

to find a neck lift in a jar as well. Some products are backed by more marketing funds than scientific studies. Components that are "firming," for example, might have some retinoid in them, but not necessarily enough to do significant firming. That doesn't mean I'm giving the OK to go online to find a higher concentration. Higher concentrations can be tricky, and super high concentrations can make your neck raw. As usual, I encourage you to see your dermatologist for the proper concentration.
There are a few noninvasive and minimally invasive treatments to improve the neck as well. Contoura Plus is used for tightening in a noninvasive way, and BOTOX® and Dysport® can also be used for banding. BodyTite™ is used for a minimally invasive option. Finally, there is a surgical option—the necklift.

Poikiloderma of Civatte is a form of skin aging from long-term sun exposure, is a dotty brown texture present on the sides of the neck. Some people have a genetic predisposition to Poikiloderma of Civatte because they are more susceptible to collagen breakdown. While there is no one golden treatment for this skin condition, hydroquinone, topical retinoid, alpha hydroxy retinol (AHAs) and lasers can all prove helpful.

A Note On Skin Sensitivity On the Neck

The neck has the second-most sensitive skin on the body. The eyelids are number one in terms of skin sensitivity. Some people cannot use the same skin care products on their neck as they do on their chest and face because they are too sensitive to certain ingredients. I am one of those people. I have a specific product for my neck and another for my eyelids because the concentration of active ingredients for normal-skin, anti-aging products have an irritating property that my skin doesn't go for. If you have sensitive skin like me, pay attention to whether the skin on your eyelids gets irritated to normal face products. If you are not sensitive, you may not have any problem using the same topical products all over. If you are curious, test a small amount of the product on the back of the neck behind the ear twice a day for a week before putting it all over.

The chest is another area that is specifically prone to skin aging from sun exposure. In fact, for many women it is the first place they show signs of aging. Nothing says aging like cleavage wrinkles. Despite its similarity in sensitivity and thinness with the neck and eyelids, we often neglect this part of our body, whether it's forgetting SPF, exfoliation or moisturizer. The good news is many treatments and procedures used to treat the face are also available to treat the chest. Resurfacing and chemical peels can help with skin texture and age spots while filler can help with wrinkles. Many topical products can be used here, too.

CARING FOR YOUR CHANGING FACE - A QUICK REFERENCE GUIDE -

When it comes to skin care, staying with the same routine for 30 years just won't cut it if you want to prevent signs of aging and maintain a youthful appearance. The minimal work needed in our 20s won't do the trick in our 40s and 50s. While everyone could benefit from getting a skin care regimen tailored specifically for them by their dermatologist, there are some basics that everyone could follow based on their age group.

- **Ages 25-29:** At 25 you still have plenty of collagen and volume, so the name of the game is to preserve and protect those assets. Most of the damage done at this age is probably from smoky environments, sun exposure, tanning and possibly some hormonal acne. Using a gentle cleanser and a light moisturizer is great for most people unless they have one of the dominant types of acne prone or very dry skin. Feel free to use a gentle exfoliating cleanser once a week, but there's no need for intense exfoliation since your skin naturally exfoliates in your 20s. Wear broad-spectrum sunscreen daily that is SPF 30 or greater and switch to a higher SPF (45 or 50 SPF) if you are going to be outdoors at the beach or on a hike. You will notice that most moisturizers contain 15-20 SPF, so depending on your skin phototype, you might need a separate sunscreen. For anti-aging treatments, use topicals that include light concentrations of retinoid, nourishing antioxidants and alpha hydroxy acids. Eat well, maintain a healthy weight, get enough rest, and try to exercise at least 3-4 times per week.

- **Ages 30-39:** If you've been using that sunscreen and eating well, you're probably in good shape. In your 30s, cell turnover slows down and natural exfoliation happens less often. Exfoliate more often with chemical alpha hydroxy acids, chemical peels, or microdermabrasion—whatever you like best. Continue using a broad-spectrum sunscreen and invest in a stronger retinoid. Continue applying antioxidants topically and talk to your dermatologist about whether you're ready for neuromodulators like BOTOX® or BOTOX®. I have many patients that receive treatment every 3-6 months. Pigmentation from sun damage may begin to show also, and if you are affected by this I recommend investing in one brown spot laser treatment in your mid to late 30s to decrease the number you have. If you have stretch marks, most have settled in and this is a good time to start treatment.

- **Age 40:** For some, hormone levels start tapering off during early 40s, resulting in dryer skin. Switch out your moisturizer for something that helps your skin retain moisture like hyaluronic acid or ceramides. Consider investing in a collagen stimulating laser each year or so, as well as a brown spot laser to keep the brown spots at bay. At this time, I usually recommend getting BOTOX® every 3-5 months as well. Continue using your broad-spectrum sunscreen, stronger retinoid and antioxidants. You may add a growth factor or peptides at this stage for more collagen stimulation. Cellulite and fat reduction procedures become popular during the 40s.

- **Age 45:** Hormone levels are declining during this time, which can cause excessive dryness for some. At this time, some women could be experience perimenopause and associated hormonal changes, which can accelerate aging. Combat and prevent further age spots with 1-2 brown spot laser treatments per year and continue BOTOX® every 3-5 months, 1 collagen-stimulating laser treatment per year, and possibly a tightening procedure for the jaw line or arms. This is also when we start to lose some volume so talk to your dermatologist about filler.

- **Ages 55-65 and over:** Skin is considered mature at this age, and you might find most of the over-the-counter products you used 10 years ago are no longer appropriate for your skin care needs. By this time most women will have entered menopause and will experience flushing, increased wrinkles, dryness and slower wound healing. Keep up with your moisturizer, as this is the primary act of defense you can do at home. Retinoids, antioxidants, peptides, and growth factors should also remain in your beauty regimen. Collagen stimulating lasers, filler, brown and red spot lasers, neuromodulators like BOTOX®, and tightening procedures may be performed more often for maximal results. Depending on how you age, this is the time when facial surgery and/or fat grafting are usually considered.

Your Cosmetic Goals: Protect, Maintain, and Repair

In the pursuit of looking your best, you will always be in a tug-of-war with time. For some, that tug-of-war presents itself as that speedy 5 or 10 minutes to put your makeup on in the morning before jamming out the door to work. For others it's the eternal struggle to get 8 hours of sleep or finding time to work out and eat healthy. For all of us, there is the sneaky way time manifests in our appearance, and that is where I'd like to help. While actually turning back the clock 20 years isn't possible (yet!). As professionals in cosmetic medicine, we are constantly researching, learning new methods, honing our skills through training and finding the best treatments and procedures available for our patients. There are currently some pretty impressive techniques that can help mitigate the aging process and keep you looking younger for longer.

In my approach to cosmetic medicine, the goal is to come up with a strategy to help you age gracefully with preventative measures, maintenance and procedures when necessary. Dermatologists and plastic surgeons have extensive training to help clients look their best. You can have your eyelids lifted, have brown and red spots reduced, have your lips plumped along with any number of other treatments and procedures. However, a lot of "looking young" is still up to you. It's about smart maintenance and making healthy decisions. For the best, most impressive results, it truly takes a combined effort between self-care and medical care. Medical care of course requires a certain medical degree and expertise, whereas self-care refers to educating yourself about what's available and understanding what you need and what is best for you. As the patient, you will always be your number one advocate and decision maker.

It's about making a lifelong skin care plan that follows three steps: protect, maintain and repair. Protective measures, as I define them, are either topical products or lifestyle habits: sunscreen, protective clothing and limited sun exposure. Protective skin care measures are also inherently preventative, so the younger these practices can find their way into your skin care regimen, the better. Ideally, protection with sunscreen and sun protective clothing should start very young, as children, while maintenance with topical creams like antioxidants and exfoliants (chemical peels and alpha hydroxy acids) should be started around age 25 or 30.

The key to aging gracefully really can be found in prevention, maintenance and repair. Together these steps can make both immediate and long-term improvements while preventing future age-related damage.

Topical Treatments and Methods to Prevent and Protect

Many women tell me how they look back on their younger self, back when they did not appreciate how good they looked at the time and wish they could go back there and enjoy it. But what if we could close that gap a bit, feel good about how we look today while also taking the right steps to look great in 10 years? If we could give our younger self advice it would probably be to take care of your skin way before you notice signs of aging. This is your first line of defense. You want to **protect** your skin from damaging environmental factors and external stressors and **prevent** rapid aging with topical antioxidants and physical sun protection (sunscreen and sun protective clothing). The sooner you adopt these healthy habits the better chance you have of combating the less glamorous parts of aging.

I grew up in Nevada, where the sun shines almost 360 days a year. I went to college in San Diego and medical school in Nevada, with an elevation of 4,500 feet. I don't have as much sun damage as some of my counterparts that arguably grew up in less sunny climates. Why? It's not because I was great at applying sunscreen when I was a kid. Instead, there are two factors that helped prevent sun damage. First, my overall sun exposure was not very high. When I was young I was a competitive gymnast and basketball player. Both indoor sports. I spent 20-30 hours a week in some sort of gym without sun exposure plus school time. If I had played soccer it would have been different level of exposure. The second decrease in load I had was honestly because I studied indoors a lot in college and medical school, therefore decreasing the amount of sun I had in my 20-30s while my counterparts were out and about. I met one of the new reps for a skin care line in my office and she could not believe the little sun damage I have on my neck and chest. I joked, spend 20 years trying to get good grades and studying and she too could have a great neckline. I am 45 and have about 15 years less sun exposure than my counterparts because of those few choices I made.

Even if you weren't a religious sunscreen user or regular exerciser in your youth, today is a perfect day to get started. In general, the more preventative and protective efforts you put in, the less intensive work will be necessary down the road, and the better those procedures will work overall when and if you do explore them. Like anything, your base health, immunity and resilience will influence your reaction to and healing from larger cosmetic investments (i.e. surgery, lasers, injections and even prescription-strength topicals). Taking preventative measures to protect your skin can start very early with sunscreen in grade school and as early as your 20s with your commitment to topical antioxidants, exercise, a healthy diet and continued use of SPF.

Topical Treatments and Methods to Maintain

It's always fun to splurge on an oxygen face treatment or luxury brand serum, but those once-in-a-while actions don't do the heavy lifting. The secret to your most beautiful skin is in your daily maintenance regimen. Your maintenance regimen always includes your baseline of prevention with sunscreen and antioxidants, but at its most fundamental level it is literally cleansing, exfoliating, moisturizing and treating on a regular basis. Maintenance methods and treatments include exfoliation treatments, moisturizers, retinoids, cleansers and most of all, consistency. Retinoids and growth factors are also included in the section, but we associate these as repair methods as well. Maintenance routines typically need a boost once you turn 30. During this time your skin should be done with all those hormonal breakouts, but it does get a little lazy with cell turnover slowing down and signs of sun damage starting to show. Maintaining your new normal and consistently caring for your skin requires these topical essentials:

- **Cleansing**
- **Exfoliating**

- Moisturizing
- Treating with retinoids and growth factor
- Consistency!

Skin care is not something you can procrastinate, and if you do, it can get expensive quickly. If you kept up with protection measures, you will likely see less damage in your 30s, 40s and beyond. Good for you! Continue using certain products while swapping out some daily products for more aggressive ones as you get older and need them. For example, you might look into more hydrating moisturizers, overnight creams and under-eye serums as your hormones shift and your skin gets drier.

No matter your budget, making room for products that stimulate cell turnover is a must. This is where your retinoid and growth factors come in. While these essentials are considered topical repair products, they are commonly used in maintenance routines to help with cell turnover once our natural processes slow down. To keep dullness and pigmentation under control, you might also consider chemical exfoliation treatments more frequently.

Topical Treatments and Methods to Repair and Improve
Despite our best efforts, signs of aging are inevitable. The good news: we have a lot of repair options available. Adding repair to your regimen can start as early as your 20s or 30s, but to what extent depends on your desire for improvements and how well you committed to preventative and maintenance measures. Repair is a choice just like maintenance and protection. Repair is available in topical, noninvasive and surgical ways. The sooner you invest in a skin care regimen that protects and maintains your skin, the better you'll look in your later years. I know this piece of advice isn't very sexy, but it's the truth.

- **Topical repair** treatment includes retinoids and growth factors. Again, these are available in over-the-counter cosmeceuticals, physician-dispensed cosmeceuticals and, prescription strength pharmaceuticals for retinoids.
- **Noninvasive** repair includes lasers, platelet-rich plasma (PRP) treatment, microneedling, light therapy, radiofrequency and chemical peels. Anything that stimulates cell turnover, wound repair and

building of collagen and elastin can be considered a noninvasive repair treatment.

- **Surgical or Intensive action** exists to help reduce signs of aging we've rightfully earned from living. For many of us, we simply did not have access to the information necessary to protect ourselves when we were in our youth. Lucky for people growing up now, they have the universe at their fingertips, literally. We simply didn't know any better, but thankfully we have advanced technology to balance some of the fun we had in our youth, like when we'd oil up to tan on the beach (sometimes with sodas and cigarettes to boot).

Knowing your skin, your genetic predispositions and the effects of your lifestyle can help you age gracefully and strategically. With the right methods and regimen, you can slow the signs of aging and feel more in control of your appearance.

The Ladder

FIVE

THE LADDER

Some patients begin considering cosmetic treatment in their 20s and 30s, while others might not consider options until their 60s. It's always a personal choice. Whenever you decide to explore treatments, navigating your path of treatment can be overwhelming on your own. You might be worried surgery will cause you to look noticeably different, or maybe you've heard horror stories about one thing or another. Remember, professional help is on your side. Your dermatologist or plastic surgeon should be your partner and mentor, there to guide you in making the best long-term decisions for your health and beauty. Throughout this book, I want to help you consider all of your options, from over-the-counter topical creams to plastic surgery.

Look, every one of us has a unique hand of cards that requires a custom-tailored treatment plan. With that said, there is a general pattern for protection and maintenance that I recommend based on your age, the age of your skin, your genetics and your lifestyle. I want to help make the process more approachable, so I've created a method of understanding cosmetic treatment from the bottom up. I'd like to introduce something I use with my own patients in the clinic every day. I call it "The Ladder."

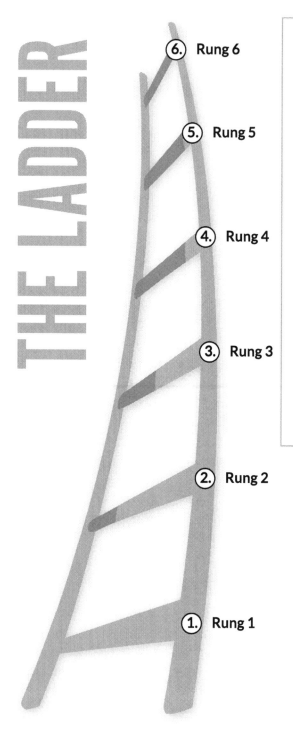

THE LADDER

6. Rung 6

5. Rung 5

4. Rung 4

3. Rung 3

2. Rung 2

1. Rung 1

Think of your options laid out on a ladder, where the options on the bottom rung are the most affordable, require the least amount of downtime, are used more often and are also comparatively the least dramatic in terms of visible change. As you reach the top of The Ladder, each rung equates to more financial commitment, more downtime, less frequent treatments and usually more risk, but ultimately more dramatic change.

Rung 1: Topicals

The first rung starting from the bottom of The Ladder holds all the topicals for prevention, maintenance and treatment. These are your household products, creams, serums and masks. These can be further broken down into cosmeceuticals, prescription-strength cosmeceuticals and pharmaceuticals. I will elaborate on these first in the next chapter.

Rung 2: Facials, Peels and More

On the second rung up from the bottom, you'll find common hydrating and nourishing practices like facials, as well as intensive chemical exfoliation procedures like chemical peels.

Rung 3: Lasers, Light-System Treatments and Other Energy-Based Treatments

On the third rung you'll find treatments relying on energy such as lasers, light and radiofrequency. These can be used to take care of marks, brown spots, hair removal and other sorts of imperfections.

Rung 4: Injectables

On the fourth rung sit the injectables like *botulinum toxin* or BTX (commonly known as the Botox® or Dysport® brand) and fillers like Juvederm® and Restylane®.

Rung 5: Minimally Invasive Procedures: Tightening, Contouring and Lifting

Near the top of The Ladder, you'll find the fifth rung, which is saved for in-office devices used by a physician for procedures such as skin tightening, cellulite treatment, fat freezing (better known by the brand CoolSculpting®) and other minimally invasive options.

Rung 6: Surgical Procedures

Finally, at the very top of The Ladder you will find procedures requiring surgery. These include tummy tucks, liposuction and the poster procedure for cosmetic surgery—the facelift.

The Ladder is broader at the bottom as topicals are the foundation to build upon and to maintain your results. As we age, we definitely want to make the first rung our baseline and continue all topicals for maintenance. The same could be said for lasers and other energy-based treatments if moderate signs of aging come to bother you. The frequency of treatments, such as lasers or injectables, may also increase, depending on your specific goals.

You can certainly be employing treatments on several rungs simultaneously, and it's possible all rungs of The Ladder will at some point be part of your regimen with time. Though, there's no correct way to use The Ladder, so to speak. You may or may not start at the bottom around age 30 and progress up. You may just want one treatment your entire life, and that's fine too. As an example, I had a patient who was about 40, a very fit lady, who worked out and carefully watched what she ate. She had four children, and after four pregnancies she had an extra bit of skin on her stomach. Her skin just did not bounce back after her third and fourth pregnancy. This area bothered her, affected the clothing she chose and just made her feel uncomfortable, but she was not interested in many other things cosmetically. My husband and I evaluated her and decided with her that she would be best suited for a mini tummy tuck. She was happy with this, had the surgery, and really did not want anything else. I, of course, put in my two cents about sunscreen and a skin check for her family. As of this day, she has not done anything on the other steps of The Ladder. One procedure was all she wanted.

I want you to know you always have the option to do *nothing* cosmetically. That's probably not something you expected to hear from me, but this is your body, your face and your life, and you get to decide what your beauty standards and norms are. While I never pressure anyone to take any cosmetic measures, I highly encourage protective steps for your skin even if you choose to do nothing more. This is because sun damage causes all those unsightly things we have talked about, and it also causes skin cancer. Skin cancer can be fatal and is to be taken seriously, so I consider protective measures to be more crucial as they are helpful beyond cosmetic purposes. I have plenty of patients that come in once per year for a skin check and nothing else. They wear sunscreen and are not interested in anything else. I tell my patients, "If it doesn't bother you, it doesn't bother me." Don't change anything you don't want to change.

Our philosophy with cosmetic medicine is to help you feel better about the way you look, and to go about it in a healthy way. The Ladder is a tool for helping you achieve your goals using our recommendations. We want to support you in taking care of yourself and investing in your beauty because you love yourself. If you prefer to do nothing because nothing is concerning you, there should never be any outside pressure. My guess is, if you've picked up a copy of this book, you have some interest in cosmetic products and procedures, so let's explore each rung in depth to see how we can best help you.

In the following sections we will look closer at each rung, from bottom to top. We will also identify the essentials as well as steps *beyond* the essentials. These sections will be categorized as *Going Further* (products) and *Honorable Mentions* (treatments).

RUNG 1: Topicals

THE LADDER
RUNG 1: TOPICALS

You will notice this very first rung on the bottom is the widest as it is the foundation for everything above it and holds all the topicals: your creams, serums and masks. This rung offers the least expensive, most accessible treatment plans with **mild** risk (assuming you are not allergic) and mild to moderate benefit if you start early. This is also the baseline that I recommend all of my patients begin with, as it will likely be part of your anti-aging regimen your whole life (if it isn't already). When choosing the right topical options for you, first know whether the product has science-backed, peer-reviewed studies confirming the outcomes. Reputable over-the-counter brands typically have information available on the website, and a focused internet search can tell you quite a lot about the effectiveness of certain products (Hello, customer reviews!). If you are using topicals to target certain skin concerns like acne scarring and pigmentation, you might want some extra guidance in the research department. You need to know whether the product has the right concentrations for your skin and is paired with complementary ingredients that will help the ingredient do its job. For example, say you're looking for an anti-aging moisturizer and you have some hyperpigmentation. While an over-the-counter product might be appealing and affordable, the concentration of active ingredient relative to other ingredients might not be strong enough to do any real repair. It would be better to see a dermatologist to help find a product with proper concentrations for your specific skin issues. We want to spend smarter, and sometimes that means spending a little extra now so you can have real benefits later.

Every single one of us is walking through the skin care aisle with a unique look and a specific set of needs. Maybe you're 35 with a darker skin tone, say Fitzpatrick Type 4 or 5 (flip to *Know Your Skin Type* for more on this), and you have noticed a recent roughness to your complexion, even though you take precautions in the sun and spend most of your time indoors. Or, maybe you just joined the 40-and-over club and feel your outside appearance does not match the way you feel inside. Or, maybe you're happily in your 50s, but you've struggled with rosacea for decades and you're now finding permanent blood vessels and redness on your otherwise light skin tone. Whatever your cosmetic goals, topical treatment can fit nicely into any regimen, so long as you know what you're using them for and the limitations they have compared to more intensive treatments.

THE TIERS OF TOPICALS

Topical products can be purchased over the counter, online, through your dermatologist or through your pharmacy. Where you get your topical treatments is very important, because it can tell you quite a bit about the overall effectiveness and what you can expect. I categorize topical treatments as either cosmeceuticals, pharmaceuticals or physician-dispensed cosmeceuticals.

- **Cosmeceuticals** are cosmetics that report anti-aging or cosmetic healing benefits and can be purchased over the counter and online. These are the products you most likely buy at drugstores or beauty department stores for daily use. They are usually an "all-in-one" product designed to treat "most women." The FDA does not regulate them, since they are specifically intended for cosmetic use. This also means they are not required to include expiration dates or concentration levels on the packaging. While there are reputable, science based and dermatologist recommended cosmeceuticals on the market, because of the lack of testing and regulation of cosmeceuticals, I highly suggest taking extra precautions when buying anything online. Make sure you're buying from a reputable U.S. or European brand you trust.

- **Physician-dispensed Cosmeceuticals** are typically offered in dermatology offices. They are tested and studied internally for effectiveness, strength and consistency by the company that produces them, but not by the FDA. These studies are sometimes published in journals and sometimes used just for effectiveness studies. These products are typically intended for daily or weekly use. Most physician-dispensed cosmeceuticals have higher concentrations than what is available over the counter. Sticking to the application instructions is crucial for physician-dispensed cosmeceuticals, as overuse can cause irritation in some cases. If you feel like you can handle more than the recommended dose, check with your dermatologist first. There's no sense wasting quality product on a hunch. Unlike over the counter cosmeceuticals, most physician-dispensed cosmeceuticals come with clearly labeled concentrations and individual ingredients for various individual reasons. I sell a separate antioxidant, separate retinoid and separate glycolic acid right out of my office. This is because each person warrants precise concentrations, not random blends of several things (which can make it much more difficult to track what's working and what's not). While I have some combo products too, combo simply does not work for everyone.

- **Pharmaceuticals** are intended for medical uses, like rashes, allergies or burns, and are prescribed by your doctor or dermatologist. They are FDA approved for specific conditions in specific doses. Your pharmacist will list the side effects when you pick them up, and they are also extensively listed on the package inserts. There are a few prescription medications that can be used for cosmetic purposes like hydroquinone for its bleaching effects and retinoids for collagen production. These pharmaceuticals help to reduce signs of aging and are either FDA approved for the cosmetic indication (like hydroquinone for bleaching) or they are FDA approved for a different indication but also have cosmetic benefits. Retinoids, for example having FDA approval for acne but can also be used for wrinkles.

There are also plenty of natural and household products you can use in your beauty routine. These would include natural toners, moisturizers and antioxidant-packed ingredients you might find in your cupboard, many of which you typically include in your diet. I have many patients who have enjoyed positive results from DIY masks, exfoliators and balms, so if this is a regular part of your routine, great! I'm a firm believer that if a product or ingredient makes you feel good (as long as it isn't harming you) then use it. There's an undeniable benefit to using certain natural ingredients that you love, whether it's avocado or coffee grounds or rosehip oil. These things make us feel good and that goes a long way in looking good. I rarely take things away from my patients (More on that later). I do warn my patients to not take household or natural ingredients too far. I had a patient once who came in to ask how to remove the blue color from her pores. As it turns out, she had read that antioxidants are good for the skin, so she had been lathering whole crushed blueberries on her face. She was happy with the results, but not the blue of her pores (Moms out there, think about how hard it was to get the blueberry stains off your toddler's fingers when they started eating blueberries themselves). We had a discussion about the plethora of available topical antioxidant creams to use instead of blueberries, how they are made for application to the face and of course, how to get the blue out of her pores (We did a few chemical peels and some exfoliation with alpha hydroxy acid at home).

If you find yourself needing a stronger antioxidant or growth factor, your dermatologist can add that physician-dispensed cosmeceutical to your natural or household product-based routine. Do you love using raw honey, olive oil or oatmeal? Then go for it! There's no harm there. However, if you're using something damaging, like washing your face with isopropyl alcohol each morning, I'm going to recommend you stop and replace it with something less drying for your skin. It should be noted that some of our favorite natural ingredients can be irritating. For example, some of my patients have had allergic reactions to oat-based scrubs and masks. Just because something is natural doesn't mean it is hypoallergenic. Use your best judgment and do what works for you.

Personally, my go-to household beauty hack product is Aquaphor®. You know the movie *My Big Fat Greek Wedding* where Toula's father sprays Windex® to fix everything? Aquaphor® is my Windex®. It comes in one-pound jars, and I need all of it. I cannot even list all of the many uses this magical ointment has, but of course I'll try: sunburn treatment, dry lips, dry skin, hand dermatitis, diaper dermatitis, curling iron burns and cuts. I even put it on my eyelids at night during allergy season. I also recommend it to patients after a skin biopsy or trauma. The caveats with Aquaphor are if you are allergic to wool or lanolin then you should use the versions that are lanolin-free, and if you are against petroleum products then you will need to look for a petroleum-free alternative. I cannot count the number of times I've had people come in who are using multiple creams, antibiotics and ointments (prescription and non-prescription) on their face, frustrated that their wrinkles are as prominent as ever and they've developed a rash. My solution: I have them stop everything for a few weeks and use only a hydrator like Aquaphor®. I check in after a month and their rash is gone and we start over with their beauty regimen. It's the same concept as your nutritionist telling you to eliminate dairy, gluten or nuts to identify an allergy. Some people are allergic to something in their multitude of products. Speaking of allergies, here's a quick word of caution: while two brands might claim the same healing or treatment benefits, it's possible you might be allergic to an inactive ingredient in one brand. Sometimes reading the back of the package can solve the issue. Common allergies include lanolin (wool), latex, sulfates and sulfites, wheat, preservatives and fragrances.

Dermabrasion

Dermabrasion is a procedure performed by your dermatologist or plastic surgeon that uses an abrasive to intentionally wound the skin to modify collagen deep in the skin. This is a surgical procedure performed while you are numb or asleep that takes a significant amount of the top layers of the skin and usually takes about 2-3 weeks to heal. This procedure is mainly used for scar resurfacing, but it also used for sun damage, acne scars and other causes of uneven texture.

When I was a resident working in the dermatology clinic, a man came in with an angry, chronic rash on his face. Why does this guy have this rash on his face? He looked like a baboon with so much swelling and redness on the face, and prescriptions only made it worse. So we started taking certain topical products away, and it started to clear up. As it turns out, he had a dramatic allergy to lanolin, an ingredient in the drugstore brand moisturizer he had been using. Lanolin is a common ingredient, and it's not harmful, except to those who are allergic to it. The prescriptions had lanolin in them also, so he was treating with his own poison for 5-6 years. Most the time if you stop everything and start over, things improve. Sometimes, nothing is better than something.

Hypoallergenic and Sulfate/Sulfite-Free Products

There's a bit of a misunderstanding about hypoallergenic products. Hypoallergenic does not mean it's better for you. It simply means it is designed to be safer for people who have allergies. This distinction is important for those who suffer from allergies and sensitive skin. According to Blakiston's Medical Dictionary, something that is "non-allergy producing" would be a preparation in which every possible care has been taken to formulate and produce a product to ensure minimum occurrence of allergic reactions. But, hypoallergenic is not "non-allergy producing." These are different. Hypoallergenic means having a decreased tendency to provoke an allergic reaction. No product is really "non allergy producing" as somebody can be allergic or reactive to almost anything. The FDA has been trying to clear up the definition of hypoallergenic by setting up testing requirements, but after some litigation it seems that this is not going to happen any time soon. So, we hope that brands are making the effort to ensure some products are "less allergic" and are labeling those as hypoallergenic. If you want to reduce the risk of an allergic reaction, I recommend sticking to products that are free of fragrance, formaldehyde, preservatives, lanolin or other ingredients that are sensitizers to a significant percentage of the population. Read labels if you have a specific sensitivity and avoid anything with your sensitizer in it. So far, no country has an official certification for a product to place the word, hypoallergenic, on labels; so we as the consumer will have to wait and read labels until then.

The Six Topical Essentials
The skin care aisle can be downright exhausting with bright colors, bold claims and dozens of brands to choose from. It's all we can do not to scream, *Help!* Once you settle your eyes on something up your alley, the product itself has a million things to tell you. While these brands are only trying to make more information and treatments available to you, it can

sometimes be less effective than they intend. For example, the all-in-one creams usually have small amounts of different anti-aging ingredients aiming to improve handful of things in a lot of people without giving too much irritation or side effects. That's a pretty ambitious task, and as the saying goes "you can't please everyone," so these products may not be customized enough for your needs. If they are working for you, that's fine, too. There are many reputable and science-based companies that create great over the counter anti-aging creams (Neutrogena®, Oil of Olay® and RoC®, to name a few). If you have tried the over the counter options and have not seen the results you are looking for, this is a sign that you need a product that is tailored to your specific needs with stronger concentrations to target the dominant aging feature that bothers you.

If you're on a budget and simply cannot afford prescription or physician-dispensed cosmeceuticals, I tell my patients to conserve money by purchasing gentle cleanser, moisturizer and sunscreen over the counter. I also encourage them to get physician-dispensed, pharmaceutical-grade retinoids, growth factors and antioxidants. If even this is out of range, that is OK. There are great over-the-counter brands. Try seeing a dermatologist and let them in on your situation. We can usually help and keep things in your budget.

For essentials like sunscreen and moisturizer, over-the-counter products work just fine for the majority of my patients. Ten years ago, I may have felt differently about sunscreen, but now that the FDA is regulating sunscreen, I feel confident recommending daily use of quality sunscreens to my patients. Moisturizer is really what works best for you; though, that can be a little confusing when a good third of the moisturizers on the shelf seem to have your name on them. You might be buying an everyday moisturizer because it is oil free, even though it doesn't do much for your fine lines. You might also have a separate daily sunscreen that's oily, but you find you don't really have much of a choice if you want to protect yourself from the sun. Talk about frustrating. Before you panic and scoop armfuls of the latest and greatest into your cart, let's identify the essential ingredients for anti-aging and beauty so you know what to look for in a product. In the following sections, we'll look at what I call the *Six (and a Half) Topical Essentials*:

Protection and Prevention
• Cleansing (the half)
• Antioxidants
• Sunscreen

Maintenance and Repair
• Moisturization
• Retinoids
• Growth factors
• Exfoliation

PROTECTION AND PREVENTION

Cleansing

We touch our face about 15 times per hour. [1] That's a lot of reasons to wash our faces twice daily.

Cleansing is the first preventative step to having clear, glowing skin. Aside from keeping your skin feeling fresh and clean, a proper cleansing routine removes daily exposures, removes makeup, and also helps other products absorb into the skin better, making them more effective. Most people spend their money on good moisturizers, serums and other leave-on products while skimping on the cleanser. (I'm guessing this logic is supported by its brief interaction with our face. It goes straight down the drain). That's fine. A cleanser shouldn't be the most expensive thing in your beauty cabinet. However, choosing the right cleanser is more about preventing certain issues, not enhancing your complexion. Finding a gentle cleanser with minimal "fluff" (i.e. scents, extra feel-good ingredients), then the cleaner your face will be. Your cleanser should be so effective that you don't need the reassurance of a toner/makeup remover cotton swipe.

Again, you don't necessarily need an expensive cleanser. What you need is a product that can gently remove sunscreen, makeup and environmental pollutants you've picked up throughout the day. I personally use a $30 cleanser by Elta MD® that lasts 4-6 months and is specifically formulated to remove sunscreen, because I use sunscreen every day. If you're really on a budget, Cetaphil® cleanser, CeraVe® cleanser, and Dove soap will work great for removing sunscreen and makeup, as will any glycerin-based soap.

If you're fond of a certain brand's product line, it's tempting to try everything on their roster—especially if the brand is featuring a new or trending ingredient, like charcoal. If your cleanser is meant to "clean your face" then make sure it does that with or without the charcoal. Most of the more expensive cleansers contain more ingredients like antioxidants or things to "soothe" or to "plump" or for "dry skin." The extras are what cost the extra money, so if you are using a regular antioxidant, you do not need a cleanser with one in it also. Many cleansers claim to be "ultra-cleansing," as in leave nothing behind. But ultra-cleansing might not always be beneficial. If your cleanser is too stripping, then you will deplete the oils in your skin and you might end up spending more on moisturizers and creams to make up for the lack of natural oils. These cleansers are also marketed as "deep clean." If you have a cream or "nourishing" cleanser, the product might contain a moisturizer that can leave residue on your face, which can clog your pores or slow the natural sloughing off of dead skin cells. Recognizing these keywords and which skin types and skin ages groups they are appealing to can help you distinguish what will work for you. Acne-focused product lines, for example, use lots of fresh, clean verbiage because one of their main demographics is younger people looking to remove gunk and acne-causing oils. Anti-aging product lines, on the other hand, target people with more mature skin by using language that signifies renewal, regeneration and moisture.

How Often Should I Cleanse?

I have patients that swear by cleansing twice a day (once in the morning and once at night) while others only cleanse in the evening. While there is such a thing as washing the face or showering too many times a day causing dry skin, I encourage cleansing every morning and evening.

People often ask me about scrubs for the face. While I am sure there are tough-skinned people that can do this every day, most of us do not need such drastic measures to exfoliate. Using a gentle alpha hydroxy acid one time a week should be sufficient for most people's exfoliation needs. Over exfoliation can cause microtears in the skin, which causes the skin barrier to become damaged. Once the barrier is dysfunctional things that did not normally irritate our skin begin to and our skin will not be able to handle the daily abuse we put it through from work, to the hot tub, to the products you put on your face. If you are exfoliating 1-2 times per week and still have texture issues this may be a deeper problem. Talk to your dermatologist and you may find you are a candidate for microdermabrasion, a chemical peel or laser. These treatments go deeper and will give you that smoother texture you are looking for. On a daily basis, we want to be gentle with our skin.

Cleansing Brushes
The mechanical cleansing brushes (and toothbrushes) have gained a lot of popularity in recent years. The brushes can range from $30 to a few hundred dollars. Some are based in studies showing that they do a better job of cleaning the skin. These are mostly the ultrasound or sonic-based mechanical brushes. The waves have been tested to penetrate the skin and dislodge more debris than regular cleansing. I do believe that this is true for both the face and the teeth (My dentist uses these for his mouth). But, I do not believe that they are an essential. They are a luxury. The cost to benefit ratio for most people is not good enough. When my patients ask about this in my clinic, I tell them what I am telling you here. I would prefer you actually get the toothbrush version first and then if still possible get the face one. Dental health is correlated with illness and longevity. The science is there so if you would like to try one of these try easing the brush into your routine. Aim for twice a week at first and then work your way up to daily. Again, I don't really recommend this as an essential, but if you have the means, it will help and by all means go for it.

Essential 1: Antioxidants
Antioxidants have been hailed as the key to a prolonged youthful appearance, for pretty much ever. [2] The fundamental role of antioxidants in the body is to neutralize free radicals and support the immune system.

Topical antioxidants protect collagen from breaking down. [3] When you apply them they grab onto the free radicals caused by sun exposure to prevent sun damage. Vitamin B3 or niacinamide, vitamin C, resveratrol and vitamin E are all used topically because of their molecular ability to penetrate the skin. Some studies have shown visible improvement of skin elasticity, erythema and pigmentation issues after 3 months of topical treatment with these antioxidants. [4]

Note: over-the-counter antioxidants may not be as effective as physician dispensed ones. When the antioxidants hit the sun, they degrade, so be careful what you purchase. Make sure the container is not transparent. Most reputable brands do this anyway. This will help you get the most out of your skin care investment

Nutritional antioxidants work to neutralize free radicals in your body by reducing oxidative stress on the cellular level. You can find plenty of antioxidant-rich foods at your grocery store, including root vegetables, fermented foods, berries and even dark chocolate (I'm talking 85 percent cocoa).

Vitamin C is most commonly known as your cold-fighting sidekick, but this powerful antioxidant also works wonders to fight skin aging. Used topically, vitamin C boosts collagen production and protects skin against early sun damage, wrinkles and other unsightly signs of aging. Look for concentrations between 10 and 25 percent. Warning: If the product contains the super potent version of vitamin C, 3-0-ethyl ascorbyl palmitate, then you only need 1-5 percent concentration. Many cosmeceuticals do not include concentrations on the label, so look for products from your dermatologist to make sure you are getting a good amount of active ingredient.

Vitamin E is one of the most common topical and oral antioxidants, as it protects against UV radiation and other free radicals. This antioxidant is the most abundant fat-soluble antioxidant present in the skin, and it may also have anti-inflammatory properties.

Resveratrol is found in nuts, berries and, the most exciting news, red wine. Studies show resveratrol protects against the harmful effects of UVB rays when used topically. Resveratrol interferes with the enzyme called sirtuins, which are known enzymes involved in the aging process. [5]

Niacinamide or vitamin B3 is a major anti-inflammatory source that reduces redness, hyperpigmentation as well as fine lines and wrinkles. Niacinamide is also extremely hydrating, though often overlooked as a "moisturizer." A few studies have shown that two percent Niacinamide is more hydrating than petrolatum and may help with the barrier function for those with rosacea. [6] This is my favorite ingredient to use in sunscreens and moisturizers in my rosacea patients.

Coenzyme Q10 is found in every cell of your body. It helps convert your food into energy and fight free radicals. Coenzyme Q10 became trendy for a while there, but at its core it is an antioxidant.

Green Tea has proved to be a potent antioxidant source, as well as an anti-inflammatory and anticarcinogenic, though it won't cancel out all those cigarettes! In order to get the benefits from green tea, you would have to drink a lot of green tea. If you are not a caffeine drinker, there are caffeine-free green teas, supplements and extracts that offer the nutritional benefits, without having to run to the bathroom every 10 minutes. There are also many topical products that include green tea as ingredient, too.

A study performed in 2008 compared multiple juices and teas for their antioxidant potential, including green tea, acai juice and many more. It found that pomegranate juice was the most beneficial for antioxidant potential. In fact, it had 20 percent more activity than its closest juice rival red wine. [7] While you're certain to get more benefit for the whole body from consuming your antioxidants, we do need them topically to directly combat sun damage to the skin. Some studies suggest higher benefits when you're getting antioxidants both topically and orally. [8]
All antioxidants get the limelight for a moment (you might notice all the praise for green tea lately), but they are just one of many sources of antioxidants. This is also why dermatologists, including myself, tend to recommend vitamin C and vitamin E, as they have been the most reliable antioxidants in skin care.

My Recommendations: While there are so many antioxidants to choose from, I recommend vitamin C and vitamin E topically, as they have loads of studies to back their effectiveness . [9] Orally, I recommend getting most of your antioxidants from great food, pomegranate juice and even some red wine.

Essential 2: Sunscreen and Sun Protective Clothing

Applying sunscreen daily is the number one method for protecting your skin against sun damage, sunspots and cancers. If you're still not wearing sunscreen, it's time to shelve your habits left over from those "we didn't know any better" days. Wave goodbye to spending scorching summer afternoons splayed out on the beach, rubbing on tanning oil and soaking up the sun. As a lifeguard I saw this every day (and I did the same thing). Now, after 20 years of diagnosing skin diseases, I simply don't go to the beach without my sun shirt, hat, sunscreen and adequate SPF. Whether you only head outside for a lunchtime walk or you work out in the fresh air from sunrise until dark, you should apply SPF before prolonged sun exposure every day.

When you're standing in front of the massive sunscreen aisle at the drugstore, it's normal to get overwhelmed. Let's break things down a bit. When I am working with my patients I explain that sunscreens can be divided into blockers and absorbers. Sunscreens work to either physically block UV rays (blockers) or absorb UV rays (absorbers), while some sunscreens do both.

So then, what causes these two distinctions? Mineral-based sunscreens like zinc oxide or titanium oxide physically block UV rays. Remember the days of the lifeguards wearing that white pasty stuff on their nose? These are physical "blockers." If you prefer physical "blocking" sunblock, now you can keep a mineral-based option without having to worry about sporting that ghost look and frightening other beach-goers. The minerals are now micronized so they rub on easier and blend in beneath makeup. You can purchase over-the-counter tinted formulations as well as affordable physician dispensed mineral based blocking sunscreens.

Many over-the-counter sunscreens use chemical filters (oxybenzone, avobenzone, octisalate, octocrylene, homosalate and octinoxate). These absorb UV rays and are what I call "absorbers." While it likely won't hurt to occasionally use the oily, waterproof chemical sunscreen you buy at the gas station on the way to the lake, anything you put on your face on a daily basis should be high quality, cosmetically elegant, and if possible, chemical

free. Many foundations and moisturizers now have SPF in them as well. Check the label for a minimum SPF 30 for day-to-day use.

Although it may seem like it, UV rays don't just disappear come fall. We are constantly exposed to UV rays, even when there's cloud coverage or it's freezing outside. Make sure to also look for broad spectrum on the label, which means it protects your skin from UVA and UVB rays. Mineral sunscreens or "blockers" are always broad spectrum.

If you're worried about missing out on beneficial vitamin D, have your levels tested with your doctor. If you are low, work with your doctor and your dermatologist to come up with a reasonable and safe strategy tailored specifically to you. Many people can get their daily dose of vitamin D through small doses of sun exposure and a healthy diet that includes lean proteins, dairy, eggs, oatmeal and orange juice. Supplementation is also a viable alternative, especially if you spend all day indoors or you have skin Type 5 or 6, or both. [10] Other candidates for supplementation include breast-fed infants (because human milk is a poor source of vitamin D) and obese people (because vitamin D is fat soluble). [11] I personally take calcium with vitamin D each day as I work mostly inside and wear sunscreen religiously.

Let's be honest, nobody really likes sunscreen. You may be fortunate and rely on a daily sunscreen you can tolerate, but ultimately we don't really like the smell, the greasiness, or the application of it. It was the joke in our house for years that my husband said I was the only dermatologist on the planet that hated sunscreen. So, when my patients tell me this as the reason why they don't wear it, I tell them all about how I hate it too, and offer the alternative of sun-protective clothing. There are many brands available now from reputable companies such as Coolibar and Solumbra that have great sun protective clothing. The designs are much more stylish than they used to be and even have wicking and cooling fabrics to help regulate your temperature. I have seen great products at our local sports store and even in some of the catalogs that are mailed to my home. I recommend a hat with a 4-inch brim and a long sleeve sun protective shirt as an alternative for my patients that hate sunscreen (and those that don't). There are ways to protect yourself, even if you hate applying sunscreen to your entire body.

Don't Forget Your Hands!

Applying sunscreen to the top of your hands is often overlooked but so, so important if you want to prevent those brown spots from forming on the hands. Commute to work? Think about how long your hands rest on the steering wheel with the sun beating down on them. I'm not saying you have to wear gloves while you drive, although I do have a patient that does this, but I also don't think it's a bad idea. If you spend a lot of time outside or commute long distances, don't skip on sunscreen. Your hands will thank you in 30 years!

Is Sunscreen Safe?

Tere is a lot of hype out there about chemical "absorbing" sunscreen ingredients being bad for you, so let's break that down. Some chemical sunscreen "absorbers" (specifically, oxybenzone) have made the top of the no-no list in the world of sunscreens because they are known to cause skin reactions and allergies. Recently, the Environmental Working Group released information linking synthetic-based sunscreens avobenzone and oxybenzone to abnormal blood levels of certain hormones in children. If the possibility of allergic reactions or negative effects of the chemicals is an issue for you, don't use them. Instead use a "blocker." As the science of sunscreens progresses, this issue will eventually be easier to manage, but until then you do have other choices if you want them.

Another circulating fear is the cancer-causing properties of sunscreens containing retinyl palmitate, an ester of vitamin A, one of the chemical sunscreens that "absorbs." First let me say that our children will be the first generation of children that are exposed to sunscreen from 6 months old through adulthood. There is real concern out there that should not be ignored as they really are the first people to wear sunscreen for greater than 60 years. We want to make sure that they are safe. In the nearly 50 years that topical retinoids have been prescribed for photoaging, psoriasis and other skin conditions, there has been no published evidence that retinols increase cancer. [12] This has been studied since the late 70s. In fact, vitamin A is often prescribed orally as a sort of chemotherapy for skin cancer patients. That being said, the Environmental Working Group Cosmetics Database rates retinyl palmitate as hazardous and potentially cancer causing because of free radicals that are generated upon sunlight exposure of retinyl palmitate. The FDA is currently investigating this. So, again, if you would like to avoid chemical sunscreens there are other options available to you now—physical "blockers" such as titanium and zinc oxide and, of course, sun protective clothing. The research will continue, and we will have firm answers soon.

There are reports that sunscreens containing titanium dioxide and zinc oxide could increase the number of free radicals in the body. Take heart. Further science has concluded that these "blockers" do not penetrate the skin. They sit on top of it. (Think about how difficult it is to rub straight zinc into your skin. It's basically impossible). However, if you have eczema or other skin disease that alter the effectiveness of the skin barrier, it might be beneficial to discuss this with your dermatologist. In addition, you can use protective clothing when your disease is flared.

Despite my high recommendation for daily sunscreen, I should note that the sun is not the enemy for most people. After all, the sun provides beneficial vitamin D through the same processes that we absorb UV rays. Because we know that UV rays cause skin cancer, we do need to be extremely careful with the amount of exposure. For optimal benefits, you must consider your skin type, duration of exposure and time of day the exposure takes place. For example, if you are skin Type 1 or 2, you are far more likely to be sunburned after 30 minutes than a person with Type 5 or 6. However, that doesn't mean you should hide under the covers all day. The experts at Harvard Medical School have said moderate exposure to the sun is much more beneficial than sudden, prolonged exposure that results in a burn. [13] In fact, the number of sunburns before 20 has been shown to have an increased risk of melanoma. [14] Other types of skin cancer like basal cell and squamous cell have more to do with the amount of sun exposure you accumulate over time. So, bottom line: some sun is good, a lot is not! Moderation is the key (Have you noticed my theme yet?). I certainly don't want you to live in a cave. Have fun in life, just be safe out there!

Picture this, my husband the plastic surgeon and I the dermatologist on our hike. He's wearing a khaki 4-inch brimmed hat and mine is white. We have large sunglasses, sunscreen on our face and neck, and our long sleeve sun shirts. The one I wear even has little finger holes so that the tops of my hands are protected. If you laughed out loud a little, so do I every time I go out. It's OK; we know that we look stereotypically ridiculous.

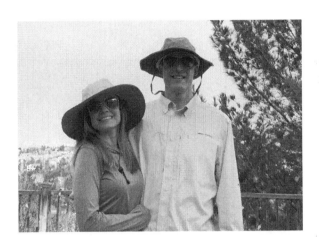

My patients often ask me what I do with my children and for my family. My family uses physical blocking sunscreens as often as we can and uses as little of the chemical absorbers as we can. That being said, if chemical sunscreens are all that is available in a specific situation I do not hesitate to use them on this uncommon occurrence. I do not believe that small doses of chemical sunscreens on an infrequent basis will cause long-term harm. But, we do purchase only physical blockers for our planned regular use and use sun-protective clothing as often as possible.

MAINTENANCE

Essential 3: Moisturization
Along with cleansing the skin, properly hydrating skin can help your overall

cosmetic goals. Skin that is consistently hydrated with moisturizer absorbs other topical products more effectively than skin covered with oil, or sebum. [15] Moisturizers are the most common therapeutic topical treatment used by dermatologists. We know that daily moisturizing is a pillar of skin health, but everyone's moisturization needs are different. There are hundreds, if not thousands, of moisturizers available, not including household ingredients or natural moisturizer recipes. So how do you choose the right one for your skin type? Refer to the aforementioned skin classifications. If you have acne-prone skin with a Glogau Level 1 (or virtually no etchings or damage from the sun) then you will need a completely different moisturizer than someone with rosacea or a Glogau Level 4. Reputable over-the-counter brands generally do a good job of labeling moisturizers for mature skin, oily skin and dry skin, but they are still pretty generalized. Once you know what level of moisturization you need, you can find a product based on the type of moisturizer.

Moisturizers do not add any water to the skin. They trap and attract the existing water from your skin or the environment. They are categorized as occlusives, humectants and emollients.

- **Occlusives** provide moisture by preventing the natural water loss of the skin from the environment by occluding the skin. Examples of occlusives include petrolatum, mineral oil, lanolin, shea butter and dimethicone. Occlusives are characteristically thick and greasy so they are often mixed with the other types of moisturizers to improve their appeal to consumers. Despite their unpleasant consistency, occlusives are one of the more effective moisturizer types on the market. Petrolatum can prevent 99 percent of water evaporation from the skin. In fact, they are well known to help treat atopic dermatitis (eczema). Applying occlusives to damp skin, or after showering, is the most effective way to use these products. Occlusives are thick and are typically designed for the body, not the face. People with acne prone skin should try to stay away from occlusives. For those who are interested, natural occlusive ingredients include avocado and rosehip oil.

- **Humectants** draw water from the deep layers of the skin to the superficial layers, allow skin to hold more water and may also pull water from the environment if you live in a climate with upwards of 70 percent humidity. [16] This moisturizer class includes honey, urea, glycerin, topical collagen, hyaluronic acid and alpha hydroxy acids like lactic acid (AHA is also a fantastic chemical exfoliant. More on that later). [17] Humectants are great for all skin types including oily and acne prone skin because they don't have any heavy oils in them.

- **Emollients** are ingredients that smooth and soften the skin making it appear less flakey. Examples include glycol, glyceryl stearate, and soy sterols . [18] Emollients can be water based or oil based and are usually used in preparations for mature and dry skin.

PEDs (prescription emollient devices)

PEDs are a newer class of moisturizers that target deficiencies in barrier function. These are prescription moisturizers that replace deficient fats in the skin. PEDs are expensive and do have some over the counter equivalents that are less expensive but in theory have fewer of the fats in them. The most commonly available over the counter versions contain ceramides. [19] **Ceramides** are the fats that are in between your skin cells in the top most layer, the epidermis. There are more than 340 known ceramides in the skin to date. Topical ceramides have been shown to decrease water loss from the skin like an occlusive does and to bring in water like a humectant. [20]

Most moisturizers that you purchase will have a combination of the three main moisturizer types. This is done to make the products cosmetically acceptable to apply but also to give you the benefits from all of them, sort of like a three-pronged approach. We intellectually understand why we should hydrate the skin if there is eczema or other skin disease, but why hydrate the skin for cosmetic purposes? Think of a raisin compared to a grape. They are really the same fruit of the same age, but one has been put in a cool moist environment and the other has been dried out. If you dry out the skin it looks more wrinkled and hydrated skin looks better, but the good thing about skin is that you can rehydrate it (which you cannot do to a grape).

If you want to apply something to your skin that will make it look good for a shorter period of time, hyaluronic acid is the key. It is a natural constituent of your own skin that holds onto water. You may know it best as an injection like Juvéderm® or Restylane®, but it is also formulated as a topical preparation. You can purchase hyaluronic acid creams from your dermatologist or plastic surgeon as a physician-dispensed product or over the counter to temporarily reduce appearance of fine lines and wrinkles. Over the counter topicals last between 1-2 hours and the physician-dispensed versions have been tested and shown to work for about 8 hours.

Do oily skinned people appear younger as they age?
In most cases, oily skin looks a little better than dry skin because the dryness makes your lines look worse. I must clarify that aging is not *caused* by chronic dryness, however dryness can make your skin appear older. While there is evidence to suggest people who have oily skin most days of the year age *differently* than their dryer counterparts. It's not necessarily true that they age better or worse.

Arguably someone with oily skin can apply more anti-aging product because the oil prevents them from drying out, which is the most common side effect of anti-aging products like retinoids. Although, because the majority of anti-aging topicals address wrinkles, we have this idea that the only sign of aging is wrinkles. As we've spoken about in previous chapters, age shows its face in many ways. From laxity to pigmentation, thinning skin to volume loss, we all age in a unique way.

Comedogenic and Non-Comedogenic Oils
In your quest for the perfect moisturizer, you have likely come across the term non-comedogenic. This simply means the product has been tested and does not form comedones (blackheads and whiteheads). It doesn't mean it is guaranteed to not give you individual pimples. However, it is especially important to look for a non-comedogenic label if you are prone to acne.

As the natural opposite to non-comedogenic, comedogenic is a classification for ingredients many people try to avoid putting on their face (which is also why most products do not include the term "comedogenic" on their packaging). Comedogenic products are not necessarily terrible for your skin; they simply have a higher possibility of clogging pores. In fact, our own sebum is comedogenic, especially for those who are acne prone. Comedogenic ingredients don't necessarily show signs of clogging right away. This can take months. This is because an individual's genetic makeup can determine how comedogenic a product is for that person's skin. Some people are just more sensitive to comedogenic ingredients than others, so it is incorrect to call a comedogenic product as *acne inducing*. This is also why products do not label themselves comedogenic. Although there is a comedogenic scale that can be used for general classification purposes. The scale is zero to V, with zero meaning the product won't clog pores at all, while V indicates there is a high likelihood that the ingredient will clog pores. (Sometimes the scale is represented as I-V, assuming anything below I is non-comedogenic).

Non-comedogenic doesn't necessarily mean oil-free either. Mineral oil and petrolatum are naturally derived, purified non-comedogenic substances that come from the ground. Both are formed from distilling petroleum, which is the liquid in rock below ground. Both have been shown to be non-comedogenic because they do not penetrate into the pores and block them to form comedones. In fact there are small amounts of both in almost all cosmetics and creams. Vaseline brand is 100 percent petroleum jelly and is tested to be non-comedogenic. Not what you would have guessed, right?

Many ingredients that happen to be comedogenic also have skin benefiting properties. Grapeseed oil is rated as a II on the comedogenic scale, contains high amounts of linoleic acid and is also a powerful antioxidant. Avocado oil is a III on the comedogenic scale and an antioxidant. Coconut oil is a common comedogenic in high demand, and it also has antibacterial and antioxidant properties. It is rated with a IV on the comedogenic scale. So the moral of the non-comedogenic story is, do what works for you!

A Quick Note On The Comedogenic Scale

While the comedogenic scale has been around for a long time, it certainly has its flaws in that it originated with rabbit ear testing. In 1989 the AAD came out with a consensus statement that if a product is not determined comedogenic on rabbit skin, it is not likely to be on human skin, and this has mostly held true. [21] Today, a lot of reputable brands do their testing on humans. These test are usually performed in a lab. We do know there is no FDA regulation on using this term (similar to other things we have seen) so we must take all claims with a grain of salt.

Researchers are working toward new models for testing comedogenicity on humans, though it is very expensive and difficult because volunteer test subjects have to be cut and risk scarring to get a human model. Most experts agree to use the comedogenic scale as a guide, but listen to your skin and your body to decide what works for you.

Oils For Cosmetic Use and Moisturization

Many of my patients use oils on their face. Whether they use them for health benefits, moisturization, or just because they like them, I don't discourage this practice unless they are having skin problems. Some of my Italian patients absolutely love applying olive oil to their face. They've been using it for 20 years and they swear by it.

There are a whole lot of oils out there used for cosmetic and treatment purposes, so when you are looking to try different oils on your face or body, first understand what you want the oil to do. Do you want better moisturization? Did you hear certain oils have anti-aging benefits?

Many naturally derived oils are in moisturizers as an ingredient and provide other benefits to the product. However, using the pure oil directly on your skin may cause breakouts if you are acne prone. We have included a list of commonly used oils rated from zero to five. If you are trying to incorporate an oil into your regimen and you have acne prone skin or have used an oil in the past and broke out, take a look at the table for alternatives with a lower number. Again, you know your skin best so if you don't have problems with coconut oil, by all means lather up.

Rating 0	Rating 1	Rating 2 & 3	Rating 4 & 5
Argan oil	Calendula oil	Almond oil	Coconut butter / oil
Hemp Seed oil	Castor oil	Avocado oil	Cocoa butter
Shea butter	Emu oil	Baobab oil	Flaxseed oil
Sunflower oil	Neem oil	Borage oil	Palm oil
Kukui oil	Pomegranate oil	Camphor oil	Wheat germ oil
Camelina oil		Olive oil	Linseed oil
Poppy Seed oil		Peanut oil	
Raspberry seed oil		Hazelnut Oil	

The Bottom Line

If you are prone to breakouts, be careful with comedogenic ingredients rated as 4 or 5 on the face or other acne prone areas like the back and chest. Remember you can be allergic to any of these oils so you should try a new oil on a small area of skin. I recommend testing on a small area of the neck 3-4 times per day for 3-4 days first before applying it to the entire face.

Face and Body Moisturizer - Where to Draw the Line

Most of us (including me) spend more money on moisturizer for the face than for the body. I personally use a face moisturizer formulated for extremely dry skin with ceramides in it, since my skin is naturally dry and I live in the desert. It costs $60 for a two-month supply. I'm thankful to have access to such great products, but even I would not put it on my body, as there are less expensive alternatives that work well. That being said, I do use it for the neck and "V" of the chest. If you are thinking about using more expensive, high quality moisturizers for the body, but don't want to go crazy, the most important areas would be the body parts that are most often exposed to the environment: the hands, forearms, the V of chest, and neck. (The same goes for treatments including exfoliants, sunscreen, antioxidants and serums, if you are able to). These are the same areas I laser for patients coincidentally: chest, neck, forearms, hands and the face. Most people don't ask me to laser the stomach as it has seen very little sun and therefore has little photoaging. For full body treatment I would recommend moisturizer daily or twice a day depending on dryness, and an exfoliating lotion with glycolic or lactic acid once every week.

Essential 4: Exfoliation

One of the best ways to improve the look of your skin is by removing the old to showcase the new. While our skin does a pretty good job shedding dead skin cells on its own, exfoliants help move the process along. Regular exfoliation improves complexion by keeping pores clean and allowing for proper oil production. Exfoliating also lets your makeup look better and creates a more welcoming environment for your topicals to penetrate the skin.

The two major methods of exfoliation are chemical and mechanical. Chemical exfoliation employs the use of hydroxy acids, retinoid, or biological enzymes derived from papaya and pineapple to rid the skin of dead cells. Common active ingredients for chemical exfoliation include glycolic acid, salicylic acid, alpha hydroxy acid, transretinoic acid and lactic acid.

Mechanical exfoliation is the physical act of scrubbing off dead skin cells with brushes and other tools or a substrate like sugar or oatmeal. If you are going to use these I prefer the electric face brushes that are specifically made to clean and exfoliate the skin. Be careful with scrub type mechanical exfoliation because too much friction can cause microtears in the skin, which can lead to uneven skin tone and may increase your chances of acne. While I don't personally recommend mechanical exfoliation with scrubs, some of my patients swear by their friction-based exfoliant, and I think whatever works for you is ultimately best. If you love using a friction based exfoliant, limit use to 1-2 times per week and avoid products with large particles for exfoliation (microparticles are better.)

Dry brush exfoliation is exactly what it sounds like—running a dry, soft brush over your skin. Originating Asia and parts of Europe hundreds of years ago, the method recently rode the detox wave into the mainstream, claiming to help with circulation and cleansing of the lymph nodes. The intentions behind dry brushing are numerous, though the science is less than approving. You can think of dry brushing as a true mechanical exfoliation, but aside from that, all other claims should be taken with a grain of salt. Also, if you are looking to use dry brushing to address cellulite, there is no evidence to back this claim, so save your money.

The Case For Separate Ingredients

When you buy a cream over the counter, you're usually buying a whole lot of moisturizer with a few active ingredients to manage a handful of skin issues mildly. While prescription-strength creams sound like the best option to get good high concentrations of active ingredients, these types of anti-aging creams aren't really covered by insurance and only some of the ingredients are available by prescription (retinoids and hydroquinone are really the only ones). Having all your necessary ingredients as separate products allows your dermatologist to personalize treatments based on your individual needs. For example, let's pretend you have acne-prone skin and need an oil-free moisturizer, but you also want to improve the look of fine lines. You need some retinoid in your regimen too. However, because your skin is extremely sensitive due to Rosacea, you may only need half of one percent of retinoid (which your dermatologist can control). Additionally, by examining your skin she can determine if you need antioxidants to help control your redness. With all this information you would likely get both a day cream and a night cream, specifically made for your skin, with the day cream that contains SPF added as well.

Sugar CAN Have A Place In Your Skin Care Routine

Don't throw away your sugar scrubs just yet. Using sugar as an exfoliant is a common practice. Sugar cane is a natural form of glycolic acid, which helps break down the stubborn protein keeping dead skin cells on your face. Raw honey is an alternative that also works.

REPAIR

Essential 5: Getting Real About Retinoids

Topical retinoids are a source of vitamin A that stimulate cell turnover, inhibit pigment and slow the breakdown of collagen. You may heard them referred to as Retin-A, wrinkle erasers, Differin® or fine line cream. Regardless of the name, all of these typically have some retinoid. Retinoids are wonderful because of their versatility in dermatology. This powerful essential improves the complexion and can help with acne, wrinkles, brown spots, texture irregularities, pore size and overall skin smoothness.

Retinoids are lipophilic, meaning they penetrate fatty (lipo) cell walls to affect expression. When you apply retinoid medication to the skin, it is taken up by receptors that work within your skin to make new proteins, chemicals, stimulants and suppressants. This process affects the changes you are looking for. The prescription topical retinoid (tretinoin) and the other prescription synthetic retinoids (adapalene and tazarotene) have been shown to clinically improve photoaged skin. [22] Retinoids inhibit pigment, increase collagen, improve texture and shrink pores.

Retinoids can be natural or synthetic, and the type available depends on whether you're getting them from pharmaceuticals, cosmeceuticals, or physician-dispensed cosmeceuticals. Each supplier and product comes with different formulations and concentrations. The prescription-strength form is called retinoic acid or retinal. Non-prescription forms are retinol, retinaldehyde, and pro-retinol (retinyl palmitate, retinyl acetate, retinyl linoleate). The body converts these into retinoic acid in the skin.

The order of strength goes from high to low: retinoic acid, retinol, retinaldehyde and then the pro-retinols. Prescription-strength retinoic acid has decades of data to support its use and should be used preferentially if possible, but over the counter retinoids (although weaker) have good anti-aging results also. While the results won't be as dramatic, over the counter retinoids might be a good place to start or a great idea if you're showing slight signs of aging. [23]

Topical Retinoids

Natural	Synthetic	Prescription	Cosmeceutical
retinol, retinyl-palmitate, retinyl-acetate, retinaldehyde, tretinoin, isotretinoin (oral), alitretinoin (oral)	tazarotene (Tazorac®), adapalene (Differin®)	tazarotene (Tazorac®), adapalene (Differin®) is now available over the counter), tretinoin (Retin A)	retinol, retinyl-palmitate, retinyl-acetate, retinaldehyde.

Retinoic acid/tretinoin is considered to be the most effective and strongest but is also very irritating. [24] If you cannot tolerate or afford prescriptions strength retinoids, retinol would be a nice close second.

Since the retinoids we are discussing are topical treatments, we have a tendency to forget that they have side effects. I recall one patient came in to see me as a medical appointment through insurance because her face was dry, red and raw in places. Before she even started to speak, I spotted it immediately—retinoid dermatitis. There is a characteristic way it looks and I have seen it many times. She told me her story, leaving out the retinoid completely. When I asked her if she was using any anti-aging medications she told me the few she was using and it did include a retinoid. I explained that the rash was most certainly a reaction to the retinoid, but she denied this possibility. After going back and forth a couple of times, and showing her a few pictures we finally agreed on the cause being the new retinoid in her over-the-counter anti-aging face cream. Remember, just because it is over-the-counter doesn't mean it can't cause side effects. I gave her a nice thick moisturizer for the evening, hyaluronic acid for topical use in the morning, and prescription-strength anti-rash medication for a few weeks. Healing from over-applying the retinoid ended up costing her twice as much as the retinoid she bought and over-used. Had she gotten that retinoid from me I would have told her to only use it 1-2 times per week and increase as tolerated. A general rule of thumb is that you want the strongest retinoid you can tolerate without significant dryness and irritation.

It's important to know what retinoid you need based on the location you are treating, your skin type, skin age and skin conditions. Start slow and realize that some skin is sensitive like the eyelids and neck, which means you may need less product or a lower concentration; or you won't need to apply it as often. Use a diluted retinoid once a week, and then increase as tolerated. For many patients, retinoids are irritating to the skin, which makes them difficult to use and almost impossible for rosacea patients or anyone with sensitive skin.

While retinoid medication is powerful, using a retinoid is a long game strategy for better looking skin. Try taking before and after photos 12 months apart. I think you will be pleasantly surprised at the changes you see. Retinoids rock, but they are not a "facelift in a jar" (Again, there's no such thing). We use retinoids to look our best at 40 or 60, not 5 years younger right now.

There are some misunderstandings and circulating myths about retinoids that have frightened people for years. Let's clear a few of these up.

1. **"Only apply your retinoid to a dry face"**
   Even the pharmacy supplied instructions say this, but I have never seen a controlled study that says applying retinoid to a slightly wet face changes the way this is absorbed. There are retinoid receptors in your skin that bind to the retinoid and neither water nor desert should affect this.

2. **"Never apply moisturizer over a retinoid"**
    This was a big no-no, even when I first started my education in dermatology. We now know that the retinoids bind to the receptor pretty quickly in your skin and although you may be diluting it some with moisturizer, it's still safe and effective if you moisturize too.

3. **"If I am not peeling it's not working"**
    This is not really true either. The retinoids work on the cellular level and the peeling is a side effect that limits how much you can use them. The peeling is why people give up on them. You want the strongest concentration and formulation that your skin can stand. I personally can only use my retinoid once per week. I cannot use retinoic acid at all as I have such dry skin, so I use retinol 0.5 percent, 1-2 times per week. I can do two times in the summer when it is more humid outside. I have my patients start with lower concentrations and formulations, and then increase in frequency once per month until they can get to every other day. If they get there I can bump them up in concentration. A mild amount of peeling when you are increasing is normal and usually improves over a month or so.

4. **"I cannot use a retinoid because I go out in the sun"**
    This is my favorite myth actually. You're not going to spontaneously combust if you walk into the sunshine and you use a retinoid. It is generally safe to wear retinoids in the sun, but they do break down in the sunlight. This is why they are packaged in opaque containers and should be applied at night. The original reports of sun sensitivity came from people walking outside and "feeling a burning sensation." Dermatologists, pharmacists, and plastic surgeons warned people of the dangerous effects of sunlight and retinoids for years, but subsequent data has shown that the MED (minimal erythema dose, or the shortest exposure of ultraviolet radiation that causes reddening of your skin) of a person using a retinoid is not any different than a person with a similar skin type that does not use a retinoid. In fact, retinoid application after sun exposure may actually be protective. UV exposure causes an increase in collagenase that breaks down collagen, but studies have shown that retinoid application after sun exposure decreases collagenase, therefore slowing the breakdown process of your beloved

collagen. [25] However, this does not counteract the need for sunscreen, so I recommend using daily sunscreen to prevent sun damage from prolonged sun exposure.

Essential 6: Growth Factors

A growth factor is a type of cell-signaling protein that acts as a fertilizer for your skin, working deep within the skin to nourish those cells, stimulate cell division, improve elasticity, and reduce the appearance of wrinkles and age spots. Growth factors give your skin that soft and supple appearance, and these same cells are at work in cell tissue and collagen stimulation. Growth factor is typically secreted naturally during wound repair, though as we age these signals slow down or become less efficient. We heal more slowly with age. In the normal healing and repair process (which occurs with damage from aging and from single wounds), skin cells and immune cells coordinate to migrate to the area and repair the area. As we age these communication signals can be disrupted and slow down. As mentioned before, you can think of aging as a chronic wound to the skin that can be repaired in ways. Topical growth factors can help keep this wound repair active after natural growth factors lose momentum. [26]

There are two main types of growth factors available for cosmetic use: plant-derived growth factors and human-derived growth factors. Science does not know everything about growth factors yet. It's a relatively new area. Plant-based are less expensive than human-derived growth factors so the normal temptation is to purchase the less expensive version. The problem with this is that if you apply a plant-derived growth factor, you may save a little money but there is a lot less scientific evidence that it works in human cells. The argument for plant-based growth factors is that the basic cell-signaling function is the same in plants and humans, so they should stimulate growth in similar ways. This may or may not be true, we really don't know yet. If in 15 years we find that the plant form is more effective than human form, or even that they are equal, I will change recommendations. For now, if you're going to spend, say, $130 on plant-based growth factors then I recommend you pay the $170 for the human growth factor because science has shown it works on humans. Here's the catch: depending on where you're purchasing your products, you won't always know if the growth factor you're purchasing is human-based or plant-based. Most over the counter versions are plant-based. However, when you purchase a physician-dispensed version, you can ask questions and be clear about ingredients, most physician offices will have both plant and human, or human only.

Is Collagen A Growth Factor?

While collagen is marketed as a growth factor, there is some controversy around whether or not it actually works topically. Collagen is an insoluble fibrous protein found in connective tissue that contributes to the strength and elasticity of your skin. [27] It's common sense to assume that if we lack something, then we need to get more of it. So is the case with collagen. There are hundreds of creams that contain collagen claiming they will reverse aging. The problem is the actual collagen molecule is likely too big to penetrate the skin and rebuild the strength of your skin. Collagen can be used topically to temporarily improve the appearance of the skin as it binds water, but there is no clear evidence that it can penetrate and be used as actual collagen or collagen precursors in the skin. There are products that say they have smaller parts of the collagen molecule that then get absorbed easier, but can the body and the skin actually take these pieces and remake collagen with them? This is unlikely, and definitely not scientifically proven to happen. When eaten in powder or pill form, collagen is digested into small peptides and these smaller peptides can be measured in blood, but I am not aware of any evidence that shows those broken-down products of collagen to be resynthesized in tissue as collagen, causing a measurable effect.

Procollagen has also been commercialized for topical application as the soluble precursor of collagen formed by fibroblasts and osteoblasts. The logic behind using this for anti-aging purposes is that the larger molecule of collagen itself has difficulty penetrating skin and that somehow procollagen would be better at penetrating. There still is no evidence that the procollagen is taken up in the correct space to then become actual collagen.

What You May Have Heard About Growth Factors

There are some concerns in the blog-o-sphere about topical growth factors causing skin cancer, since many growth factors stimulate cell division. In fact, there was an attempt at a class-action lawsuit in 2015 claiming that these topical growth factors increased skin cancer. The suit did not go far as it is difficult to prove that growth factor itself has increased skin cancer. We do know from various studies going back about 18 years that growth factors do help with the signs of aging, and newer forms are only becoming more effective. [28] But, is the concept that they can cause skin cancer plausible? Most dermatologists and scientists report they have not seen a case and do not believe that this actually happens in real life, but that it could be theoretically possible. Remember, modern medicine is only 100 years old, we don't know everything yet. Back in college I learned that my roommate's mother had received radiation to her face in the 1940's for acne. At the age of 50 she had numerous skin cancers already, more than would be expected from her sun history, and she had none in the areas that were not radiated. Her current physicians told her it was from the radiation she had received as a teenager. Something that science thought was helping her ended up hurting her years later. We now know that radiation should not be used in this way and that it does increase cancer. So, if you are concerned about this as a remote possibility and want to stay away until there is firm data one way or another, there are alternatives that are not growth factors that offer great results to add to your regiment—peptides. I personally use peptides and a growth factor on my face twice a day, but you should discuss this and your individual risk factors with your dermatologist.

Going Further

Outside of the topical essentials, there are at-home methods, professional treatments and standard procedures that can help you achieve certain goals more effectively. I do not consider them "essentials" for different reasons. Some are not as safe, others are just not practical for daily use and some are just not a great bang for your buck. But, I do get asked about them often so let's review a few hot topics.

Microdermabrasion

There have been a number of times where a patient has come to me asking about "dermabrasion" when they really mean microdermabrasion. While these terms sound pretty close, it's important to know the difference so you can manage expectations and get the results that are closest to what you're after.

Microdermabrasion is a mostly painless, noninvasive procedure performed by an esthetician that uses sand, diamond or a mechanical exfoliation device to exfoliate the superficial layers of the skin and produce cell turnover. This is an excellent procedure for exfoliation. After a period of regular treatments, microdermabrasion may also help a little with fine lines, wrinkles and large pores. Unfortunately those with severe acne, scarring or deep wrinkles will not have a lot of benefit from this procedure. Microdermabrasion is perfect for those looking for regular preventative treatment and mild maintenance.

I have seen the term, dermabrasion, used for topical at-home treatments, and I would like to clarify that those devices and products are micro-microdermabrasion (i.e. basic exfoliation), not dermabrasion.

Toners

Like many people I talk with, you might also remember the burning, astringent "toners" of old. You might remember dousing a cotton ball with something that looked and smelled like rubbing alcohol and then slathering it all over your face, neck and chest. Those high-in-alcohol "toners" are all but out today, thankfully. Toners are meant to hydrate, not zap your skin of moisture like pure alcohol would. In addition to hydrating elements like hydrogen and oxygen, many toners now include antioxidants and anti-inflammatories. Toners are used to deliver your skin a swipe of hydration and remove dead cells from the skin's surface, giving you that *glow* you're after. Toners also help you achieve the right pH balance. Let's dive into that a bit.

Studies show a healthier skin is closer to 4.7, or slightly more acidic; though, popular assumption claims a healthy skin pH sits between 5 and 6. Maintaining a healthy pH balance can help prevent dry skin, breakouts and other skin issues. Washing with harsh soap and even some tap waters can elevate the pH of your skin for six hours. Using a soap free cleanser or a toner can bring the pH of the skin closer to the optimal number. There are so many toners available you do have to monitor what you are buying, making sure to avoid alcohol-based toners. One of the primary goals with pH balancing is to make your skin more receptive to nourishment. That simple pH change and manipulation can help certain medications penetrate better. Toners have gotten popular because people love to see how much dirt their cleanser missed. My recommendation: buy a high quality cleanser and you won't need a toner to remove dirt, just to balance pH. If you want a toner, then choose something with low alcohol content from a reputable company, preferably from your dermatologist.

Cleansing With The Right Water

There is some data to suggest that certain types of water can disrupt the pH of the skin. In some parts of the world the pH of the tap water is VIII, and there is increased worry about using hard water or well water for cleansing of the face. I am of the opinion that tap water is just fine unless you have a problem with significant dryness, acne or another facial condition. Yes, there are irritants and metals in hard water, but the side effects are minimal. Some people might experience dry skin, and it's possible to irritate and worsen atopic dermatitis; but if you don't have this problem then it is probably not an issue for you. If you do suffer from chronic irritation or dermatitis, using bottled water to wash the face could be worth a try to see if it can help you.

Alcohol And Your Skin

When we hear the words alcohol and skin in the same statement, it's common to cringe. But what is alcohol, and is it all-terrible for your skin? It's not so black and white.

There are several different types of alcohols: solvents, emulsifiers, antiseptics, preservatives and pH balancers. The main three in skin care are simple alcohols, fatty alcohols and aromatic alcohols. Simple alcohols are used for the antiseptic effect and come in forms such as methanol, ethanol, isopropyl alcohol, and denatured alcohol. This type is the one that dries out the skin and is the main type of alcohol that we don't like.

Other types of alcohol that are OK as an ingredient include the non-drying types of fatty alcohols including sterile alcohol, oleyl alcohol, isostearyl, myristyl, lauryl, cetearyl and caprylic alcohol. Lastly, there are the aromatic alcohols like benzyl alcohol. Aromatic alcohols give products their fragrance.

Next time you look at the bottle, look a little closer than the word alcohol before tossing it. Most of the time people are referring to putting isopropyl alcohol on the face. This alcohol causes a quick drying and degreasing effect, causing the skin to feel tight and clean, but it also causes dryness and microscopic erosions of the skin. The dryness and erosions make it harder for those treating acne to stick with the routine as acne products cause some dryness and irritation also. There is some evidence that alcohol also causes cells to die. [29] The death of the skin cells clogs pores and can increase acne. However, this is controversial, as it has never been shown in real life, only in a petri dish.

There's a circulating myth that, because of alcohol's drying properties, it can cause overproduction of oil, resulting in worsened acne. I don't think this is true. I have not found any scientific evidence that oil is increased in any measurable amount after using alcohol to the face.

After all of this being said, if I had a patient who came to see me and said alcohol was the only thing that works for them or the only thing they could afford, I would not say no. Why? No. 1: it doesn't cause cancer or any significant damage besides dryness. No. 2: if it works for them, and I mean really works, then it works for me.

For the Budget Conscious

I'm not big on recommending brands, but I do recommend Oil of Olay®, RoC® or Neutrogena® to many patients with mature skin when all pharmaceuticals and physician-dispensed cosmeceuticals are unaffordable for them. RoC® contains retinoids, Neutrogena® is sufficient for acne, and Oil of Olay® is a solid product from a reputable company that contains peptides.

So with some scientific evidence backing peptides and all the great things they can do, you're probably wondering why I have not categorized them as an essential. The truth is peptides are still a controversial topic and can be quite expensive. So, use the essentials first and if there is room in your budget and on your bathroom counter add the peptides in. Peptides have the best chance of working if they are put in a stable cream that is made by a reputable company. My recommendation is to use one dispensed by your dermatologist if you are considering using one.

Peptides

Twenty years ago, scientists and doctors never thought peptides would have a place in our anti-aging regimens. Since the turn of the century, synthetic and natural topical peptides have gained a top spot in our anti-aging toolkit. While the peptides are certainly flying off the shelves as scientists find more certainty in their effectiveness, there are fewer studies on peptides than on the six topical essentials outlined previously. If you have to choose between new products like peptides and traditional products like retinoids, moisturizers and antioxidants, make sure to use the most scientifically backed essentials first and fill in with peptides when you can. From a molecular standpoint, peptides are larger than the previously confirmed size of molecules able to penetrate the skin. So there is more research to be done before we can consider peptides a topical anti-aging essential. Some early evidence suggests that peptides can penetrate or act as penetration enhancers and increase collagen.

Fat is Back! Lipids and the Skin

You might have heard new buzzwords like "lipids" and "ceramides" popping up in beauty blogs and in the skin care aisle, and while the science behind these chemicals in skin care is fairly new, there is something to be excited about in the field of moisturization and barrier function. A lipid technically means a chemical molecule or compound that is not soluble in water. Fatty substances like animal fats and plant oils are made of lipids. There are various types of lipids, such as fatty acids, phospholipids, glycolipids, cholesterol, triglycerides, waxes and steroids. They affect skin barrier function and play an important role in cell-to-cell signaling. Because epidermal lipids are so crucial to the skin's barrier function, the skin barrier is often referred to as the lipid barrier. Almost all moisturizers (except for some oil-free products) contain barrier repair ingredients, especially those for dry skin and sensitive skin. Barrier repair ingredients may also work by providing a temporary protective film over skin. A damaged barrier allows water to escape more readily because it is more 'porous.' That's where your occlusive moisturizers typically come in.

Our skin contains quite a list of sebaceous lipids (squalene, triglycerides, free fatty acids, wax ester, cholesterol and cholesteryl ester) and extracellular lipids (ceramides, cholesterol and free fatty acids). The extracellular lipids are the ones people are thinking of when they see lipids and skin care, as they are part of the top layer of the skin. Changes in the concentration of these make skin dry or cracked. Sebaceous lipids are secreted from oil glands called sebaceous glands. Their job is to moisturize and protect our skin. Imagine a brick wall. The bricks are the cells of the skin and the glue in between is the lipid.

Ceramides

Ceramides are a type of extracellular lipid that live in the epidermis. Like cholesterol and free fatty acids, ceramides are one of the primary lipids that help to maintain the health of the skin barrier, or stratum corneum, and keep your skin all plump, smooth and hydrated. You can think of these lipids like a glue holding skin cells together. Extracellular lipid content of the skin is directly related to barrier function, and if you apply ceramides topically it has been shown to improve injured skin that is dry or flaky. Ceramides make up roughly half of the lipids in the skin barrier, which is why changes in the amount of ceramides in the skin barrier are linked to skin conditions like atopic dermatitis, redness and itchiness. The lack of ceramides makes the skin barrier more prone to environmental pollutants and pathogens.

Around age 30 the amount of naturally present ceramides drops pretty significantly, so I'm not surprised that many patients have been asking about them. I have ceramides in this section because they are often found in higher end cosmeceuticals. While not technically a moisturizer, these lipids have become an increasingly popular addition to moisturizers. Also, naturally occurring ceramides are very expensive to source, so synthetic or plant-derived ceramides (phytoceramides) are becoming increasingly popular. Like the logic that upholds the popularity of plant-based growth factors, phytoceramides have similar chemical properties as human-derived ceramides, so in theory they may work just as well, though the verdict is still out.

While ceramides are not considered an essential, if you have room in your budget, I do recommend using them after age 30. Studies show if you apply ceramides for 21 weeks, your skin barrier will improve. I use a ceramide-based moisturizer each night for my face and eyes.

 What About Ceramide Supplements?

Some phytoceramide supplements are available, using the logic that the body absorbs them into the bloodstream, which then nourishes the skin. Many of these phytoceramide supplements are derived from rice. Like oral collagen supplements, there isn't much evidence to support that phytoceramides taken as supplements can be absorbed or make a difference, so stick to topical ceramides.

Cholesterol

If you take cholesterol-lowering agents like statins, you might have noticed your skin has gotten dryer. That's because cholesterol is also in the skin so when you lower it in your body, you can see the changes on the outside too. Cholesterol in skin naturally decreases by 40 percent by age 40, so the added medication intensifies that. Topical moisturization works to help keep some cholesterol in the skin, but I also recommend looking for a cream with cholesterol in its ingredients. Look for topicals with wool extract or lanolin extract (unless you're allergic) in them, since cholesterol is derived from these emollients.

FACE MASKS

Masks are one of those popular treatments that are well marketed as an essential, but I would argue otherwise. Masks are usually put on in a pampering state of mind, maybe combined with a bubble bath and candles, a glass of wine and an audio book. There's no doubt in my mind that masks, in this way, are very much part of a proper self-care regimen. Masks, specifically spot-treatment masks, are also helpful in circumstances where a little extra TLC is needed—like when you wake up with an angry pimple, or after traveling. However, I do not consider masks as an essential skin care treatment, they are more of a luxury.

Just like lotions, creams and serums, a mask is ultimately another way for your skin to absorb essential nutrients. If you want to get the most out of your masks, regular exfoliation techniques can help nutrients penetrate the skin better.

There are hundreds and hundreds of facemasks out there. There are masks for treating acne, masks for moisturizing, masks for drying skin out, mask for exfoliation, overnight masks, and under makeup masks. There are mud and clay varieties and then there's cream or honey based home masks. There are so many masks out there that multi-masking has become a thing, which, if you're a mask person, is a wildly effective way to tackle several issues at once. Sometimes you need a little moisture here and a little acne spot treatment there.

If you love masks and consider these an essential, I have a few tips for masking effectively.

1. Know what you want treated and find a mask with active ingredients for those specific issues.
2. Always read the label carefully and follow the directions. If it says keep on your face no longer than 20 minutes, abide by their recommendations.
3. If you have sensitive skin or if you are using this product for this first time, I suggest testing the product by dabbing a bit on the skin behind your ear or near the inside of your wrist. Labels typically indicate whether or not the product is suitable for sensible skin and provide alternate directions.

Masks are alike to the essentials in the sense that the quality and concentrations can vary greatly depending on where you're getting them, or if you're making them at home. Masks do not necessarily work better than other topicals to achieve what you're looking for it to achieve. When choosing the right masks for your skin issues, you want to know what it is you are trying to treat. The best masks will have essentials in them, like antioxidants and moisturizers.

Reputable cosmeceutical companies are improving their mask products all the time. There's nothing wrong with them, but if you only have the budget or time for your six essentials, I say don't worry about adding masks into your routine unless you absolutely love them. I won't stop you. Think of them as more of a luxury than an essential.

Honorable Mentions
With all new products, I encourage my patients to know what they're goal with the product is and make sure this is in line with the claims a product is making. The things that flash in front of you that you don't hear about in a year are probably not the things you want to adopt. The things that have been relatively permanent in the dermatological landscape (retinoids) is something you should spend money on. At a certain point some of the flashes will become permanent, so if you just wait for the date to come out, it will likely be a better investment. Put your effort and money into the permanent ones.

If you are employing all six essentials in your routine, you've tried some of the products in the *Going Further* section, and you have a little extra in your budget for something new, then there are a few "Honorable Mention" products I would recommend experimenting with.

Probiotics and Prebiotics. Probiotics became popular with those yogurt commercials endorsed by Jamie Lee Curtis, and for good reason. Probiotics have recently been studied in depth, and scientists have found these "good bacteria" have anti-inflammatory properties, aid in immune health and promote healthy skin and hair. [30] The goal with probiotic skin care products is to increase the good bacteria in the microbiome layer of your skin without having to down quarts of yogurt. The logic here is that, like antioxidants, you can apply probiotics to the skin directly while also including them in your diet.

Although probiotic skin care doesn't have enough science behind it for me to recommend it as an one of the six anti-aging essentials—or a *Going Further* product—there is no science to say it is harmful either. [31] Before investing in a probiotic cream, know what your goals are. Do you want to use it for anti-aging, anti-inflammatory or overall health? Pick your products based on that goal.

Makeup Removers
Makeup remover is a vehicle to get rid of makeup, it does not need to be expensive, it just needs to work and not do harm to the skin. When I tell my patients I often use good old Dove soap to remove my makeup, they're floored. While I spend decent money on my cleanser, I personally think pricey makeup removers are not worth the money. They typically don't have any healing or anti-aging properties in them because the goal is simply to get the mascara off. If you love wearing makeup, all you need is a gentle cleanser or the oil of your choosing to wipe your eyes clean.

Whatever you decide to use is OK with me, with one exception: if you have sensitive skin you should be careful, as the skin around the eyes is the most sensitive skin on the body. Many makeup wipes or make up removers have chemicals and preservatives that definitely get the makeup off but may be irritating to the skin around the eyes. I get the convenience of them though.

If you're traveling or camping, then using these once in a while isn't the end of the world. But, in general I recommend more gentle options when available.

Beauty Supplements

Ingestible beauty has recently found itself on the shelves at beauty and skincare retailers. These supplements, which typically come in powder form, are definitive of the modern market. Today, wellness and beauty are one in the same, so it is no surprise these beauty supplements are flying off the shelves. Packed with "beautifying superfoods" and appealing to our on-the-go lifestyle, adding these to your diet is thought to be a quick and easy way to give your skin all the nourishment you need. If you look at the ingredients in these powders, you might notice there are loads of antioxidants, vitamins and minerals in them. The beauty powders are basically replacing capsule vitamins and some even claim to replace full meals, depending on the type of powder you get. With that said, I am a firm believer that you can get all of your nutrition from a diet rich in vegetables, good fats and lean protein. But, I also know what it's like to be on the run. These ingestible beauty products are not an essential. They should be considered a source of additional vitamin, antioxidants and minerals. If you plan on taking a supplement at all, try to stay away from the brands and products that contain a lot of fillers or binders in the product, as these are definitely not necessary.

Risk–Benefit–Cost

Risk Level:	Benefit Level:	Cost:
Mild	Mild/Moderate	$

Risks and Precautions

As an overview, the primary risks and precautions for topical products involve the credibility and concentration of the products. Most over-the-counter products will not harm you, unless you have certain allergies, or you use more than the product calls for. Follow the directions provided with the product, be cautious when self-treating and with online purchases; and when in doubt, see your dermatologist.

RUNG 2: Facials, Peels and More

SEVEN

THE LADDER
RUNG 2: FACIALS, PEELS AND MORE

While Rung 2 makes for a relatively short list of items, there are a few common practices within it that I'm asked about quite often. The first group of procedures includes facials -- the common ones like many of us have enjoyed at day spas -- as well as more atypical entries that get a lot of chatter because of their unconventional ingredients and treatments, like the "vampire facelift." Overall, the treatments in Rung 2 provide mild/moderate results, with even better results if you receive treatments consistently over time. Since these treatments include stronger exfoliation methods and ingredients, you can also expect mild/moderate risk as well.

Facials
Remember when I said I've had very few facials, and how I said you will not spontaneously combust without them? Well, this is true, but there are benefits to facials that work in conjunction with your topicals for maintenance. They are not essential necessarily, but they have their place for many women. The benefits of facials vary depending on the products used and the technique and experience of the esthetician. A certain facial has a standard line of products used based on what it is supposed to do. As an educated consumer, you can get the most out of a facial by going to someone with experience that is ideally located in a dermatologist or plastic surgeon's office. This type of esthetician usually has the most experience, the most tools available to her or him, and the best product lines and services to offer you.

- Antioxidant
- Oxygen
- Enzyme
- Exfoliating
- Hydrating
- Anti-aging
- Acne
- Deep Cleansing

Depending on your dominant aging features you and your esthetician can choose facials best suited for your skin. Facials can be combined with topicals, peels or other treatments to maximize benefits for your specific skin.

Facials Are Important For Those With Acne

In acne patients I have found that acne facials can be cleansing, decrease medication use, and improve the appearance of acne and overall self-esteem.

Facials Involving Pearls and Other Sea Ingredients

If you're into skin care, chances are you have a few products that have sea-derived ingredients like algae, kelp or pearls. During my surreal boutique experience in San Francisco I sampled products with crushed pearls in them. They can be put on topically or taken internally and have been used in China for many years. Pearls contain calcium, minerals, amino acids and magnesium, which are great things for the skin. Pearls are also used as a topical "brightener," which should be thought of like a highlighter or mineral makeup rather than a bleaching product. Pearls have been advertised to contain antioxidants that boost superoxide dismutase, an antioxidant enzyme that can stimulate the generation of collagen if taken orally. Pearls are no doubt a great source of antioxidants, calcium and minerals when taken orally, but there is no scientific evidence to support the claim that it helps produce collagen.

As far as other sea ingredients go, most help with anti-aging because of the antioxidant properties, so kelp it up if you are so inclined.

Vampire Facelift and Gold Facials

You may have heard in the news about a new skin care trend called a vampire facelift or vampire facial. The vampire facial was heavily covered in the media after it was known that Kim Kardashian had one. [1]

The technical name for a vampire facial is *platelet rich plasma facelift* or *platelet rich fibrin facelift*. This is not actually a surgical facelift, but an in-office, facial rejuvenation procedure. It is named the "vampire" facelift because it involves the patient's own blood drawn from their arm, spun, and then applied to the face in order to stimulate collagen, therefore "lifting" the skin. Some people use this platelet rich plasma technique with laser or other fillers including Juvéderm® and Restylane® for a more noticeable result.

There is another trend in some of the higher end salons in the U.S. and among celebrities called a gold facial. This trending facial is a type of spa treatment that includes the application of a facial mask made with 24-karat gold foil. These facials are marketed to have benefits for its improvement in skin texture, tone, appearance, redness, elasticity, wrinkles, dark spots and hydration because of the softer composition of the precious metal. Unlike the vampire facial, the gold facial has reportedly been around since the days of Cleopatra, who is rumored to have done it every night to maintain her beauty.

I completely understand the desire to pamper yourself like Egyptian royalty, but it might be out of reach for most of us. These facials can cost between $400 and $1,200. The facials that use 24-karat gold often also use hyaluronic acid, bee venom, massage or antioxidants. Most dermatologists would agree that the hyaluronic acid or antioxidants you received with the gold at your facial had just as much benefit than the actual gold did.

While the vampire and gold facials are enjoying a hyped up status in the media, you don't need to pay big bucks for this exact process to see the great benefits. In fact, there are several other options that incorporate the same science. You can get results without the hyped brand name that your local superstar got this week. Ask your provider what is available to you locally and what works for your specific needs.

If you do opt for the vampire facial, we encourage you to apply the questions we've provided as you work to become your own advocate. No matter where you receive the facial, do not lose sight of the nature of the procedure. They are drawing your blood. Blood can harbor Hepatitis C, HIV and other pathogens. Remember to take note of hygiene and safety details.

- Are they using a single-use needle?
- Did they throw it in the sharps container afterward?
- Do they have training in blood borne illnesses?
- How do they clean the equipment?
- Do they know what they don't know?

When there's blood or bodily fluids involved, professionals should be credentialed in the proper hygienic process of handling these fluids and the tools that come in contact with them. I know how much my autoclave (high heat steam sterilizer) at my office costs to purchase and maintain, but it is necessary to ensure sanitization and patient safety. Always check with your provider to make sure they are taking necessary steps to ensure the sanitization and safety of their tools, and do not have procedures done anywhere that do not abide by these basic safety and hygiene standards.

Chemical Peels

A chemical peel is a chemical exfoliation that uses a solution (lactic acid, glycolic acid and salicylic acid are some common ones) to be applied to the skin commonly on the face, neck or hands, but can be applied to other areas of the body. A chemical peel helps to improve complexion, uneven skin tone and signs of aging. The science is pretty straightforward. Chemical exfoliation causes old skin to slough or "peel" off, revealing a new layer of skin beneath. Chemical peels can improve hyperpigmentation, mild scars, fine lines and age spots. With salons and board certified dermatologists alike recommending chemical peels, there's some things you should know before scheduling your first peel. First off, there are three basic types of chemical peels categorized by the depth of treatment.

Superficial Peel uses a mild acid like alpha hydroxy acid to gently exfoliate the top most layers of the skin. This method is used for mild skin pigmentation, rough or dull skin complexions and as a general skin refresher and is usually performed by a licensed esthetician. Recovery from the superficial peel can take anywhere between 1-7 days and will likely cause some mild redness and fine peeling. However, it is typically safe to wear makeup the following day. I recommend wearing sunscreen afterward as protection for the new baby skin.

Medium Peel goes a bit deeper with the help of stronger and higher concentrations like glycolic or trichloroacetic acid. Jessner's solution is also used for medium peels. A medium-depth peel is typically used to treat everything targeted in superficial peels as well as wrinkles, moderate skin pigmentation and acne scarring. It is usually performed by a high-level esthetician with physician supervision or a provider like a nurse practitioner, physician assistant or physician. In some cases you can also use this peel to treat actinic keratosis or pre-cancerous growths. Medium peels usually require 5-7 days of recovery time and involves good cleansing, application of ointments and, at times, oral antiviral medication. Redness and swelling continue for up to 48 hours. The skin will peel off within the 5-7 days revealing healthy, fresh skin with fewer sunspots. The full collagen stimulation may take up to 9 months. If you are doing this type of peel for acne scarring or wrinkles, multiple treatments are usually required and results can be expected after a few months. Makeup is safe to use about a week after the procedure.

Deep Peel stays true to its name. The deep peel treats the same problems as the superficial and medium peels, but goes deeper for deeper scars, and moderate to severe lines and wrinkles. The deeper peels penetrate to the middle layers of the skin and usually use phenol. This peel should only be done with experienced physician's hands, as there are some cardiac risks and you need physician supervision. Deep peels take 14-21 days to fully heal, and redness may last a few months afterward. With the invention of lasers, the deep peel option is rarely done anymore, but it is worth knowing about.

If a chemical peel sounds like an appropriate treatment for you, then a full consultation and examination from your dermatologist or plastic surgeon will be the next step. While it is all too easy to walk in somewhere and schedule a peel (or buy an online one to do yourself at home), I highly advise you to get examined first. Typically, chemical peels must be toned down for patients with darker skin. They it can cause hyperpigmentation or discoloration. I once had a patient who came to me with dark, striped lines across her face, looking for a solution. She was a skin Type 4, which means Hispanic type with brown skin; and therefore, she was more susceptible to pigmentation. She had purchased a dark spot-correcting peel online. After she applied it to the skin, she developed blisters on her face, causing these dark streaks across her cheeks. Once we looked closely at what happened, the peel was not made in the U.S. The box wasn't sealed and she bought an acid way too strong for over-the-counter use. It was 50 percent glycolic acid. With skin Type 4, she needed a much lower concentration than she purchased. Using this product on her skin caused burns with similar intensity to blistering sunburns. Even if it had been made in the U.S., not all products are regulated during transportation. It could have sat in a truck from Massachusetts to California in a 175-degree environment, growing bacteria during transport. With prescriptions and physician-dispensed cosmeceuticals, regulation is standard. A certain percentage of products are pulled and randomly tested to make sure they are safe, active and not contaminated. If I use a product from a reputable physician dispensed company, I know that it is tested randomly, regularly and to a safe standard. I stand behind their products. I encourage you to treat your face and other parts of your body with care. Do not buy from unknown companies online. Stick with the tried and true brands that stand behind their products.

DERMAPLANING, MICRONEEDLING AND MORE

Dermaplaning is the process of using a special scalpel at a 45-degree angle to the skin to remove dead skin cells and hair. Dermaplaning is used almost like a chemical peel to remove the surface layers of the skin and leave smooth new skin underneath. It has the benefit of removing hair also, which is why some people may choose it over a chemical peel. There isn't any significant collagen stimulation or deep change, but it does give a nice glow to the skin and allow medication to penetrate better and makeup to lay nicer.

Dermaplaning can be performed by a qualified esthetician, which is defined differently depending on which state you're in (In Nevada a medical director must supervise the person performing the treatment). This procedure is completely safe for pregnant or nursing patients because it is a 100 percent mechanical procedure. No chemicals needed.

Microneedling, also known by micro-penning or by the popular brands Dermapen® and Derma Roller®, is the process of puncturing small holes in the skin with a roller, a pen, or a stamper to stimulate collagen production, reduce signs of aging and improve appearance of scars. Microneedling stimulates collagen, softens wrinkles and creates micro

Treat Yourself - At Home Microneedling Devices

At home microneedling devices are becoming more popular for smaller, more frequent treatments. Specifically, the dermaroller can be considered as a sort of next step for better penetration of your serums and topicals used at home. This is also a good option if you are looking for a milder alternative to a formal microneedling treatment at your dermatologist's office. While less intense, the at-home device may be able help stimulate collagen production while also improving penetration of your other medications and serums. While buzz around these devices has seen a major boost lately, this device has actually been around for over 15 years. While microneedling has been praised for treating acne scars, fine lines and other signs of aging, the effectiveness of this treatment depends on the size of the needles being used, the depth of penetration and the frequency of use. When the punctures are deeper and/ or wider, you stimulate more collagen and your skin care products will be transported deeper into the skin for maximum benefit. The at-home devices are typically equipped with needles no longer than 1 millimeter, and the science behind this small of a needle is lacking. Dermatologists typically have devices with needles as long as 3 millimeters and commonly use a topical numbing agent to help you tolerate the procedure. In a 2009 study, roughly 94 percent of patients saw improvements in acne scars with treatments using 1.5

(continued)

millimeter needles. The size of the needles will also determine how frequently you should be treating yourself at home. Most of the at home devices are safe to use 2-3 times per week, and if you have sensitive skin you might find once a month is plenty of puncturing for you.

My reservations with at-home microneedling are rooted in risks associated with at-home puncturing of any kind—infection. A good rule of thumb for at-home devices of any kind is to abide by the same hygiene principles your dermatologist would in a formal treatment. We either autoclave or dispose of any material that has penetrated the skin of a human. Do not lose sight of the fact that at-home devices penetrate the skin, should never be shared and should be cleaned well or replaced. The other thing to remember is that you do have bacteria on your skin, more potentially if you have acne or rosacea. If you plan on purchasing an at-home device, do not use it on inflamed skin or active acne. If you have cystic acne, I recommend waiting to do any treatment until it is fully clear. Under no circumstances should you share the device with someone else. Even if your mom is dying to try it, kindly show her where she can buy her own online. You can easily spread terrible diseases like hepatitis by sharing. Follow the instructions provided with your at-home device on cleaning and replacing parts.

channels on your skin for creams and serums to work more effectively. The tiny pinpricks inform your body to send collagen to repair the damage, which improves overall skin texture. Microneedling can also be used to treat fine lines, acne scars, texture irregularities and traumatic scars.

Weighing Options: Microneedling Or Deep Chemical Peel?
Can't decide between microneedling and a chemical peel? These are both cost effective treatments for aging, but really do treat different things. It

can be difficult to gauge benefits just by reading about them. Typically I look at the patient and discuss with them what they are looking to improve and help them choose based on budget, downtime and goals. In my experience, microneedling will stimulate collagen a little better than a peel (unless you opt for the super intensive chemical peel performed in the operating room where you are put to sleep for the procedure; but few people do those anymore). Chemical peels will improve surface issues like sun damage, and work better for brown spots. In general, chemical peels are less expensive. Downtime is also a factor. If you need to get back to work, a superficial microneedling would be the way to go. This procedure requires a day or two of irregularities. A mild peel by your esthetician will have a few days of mild peeling, whereas a dermatologist-performed TCA (trichloroacetic acid) peel can be a week of exfoliating/peeling.

Risk–Benefit–Cost

Risk Level:	Benefit Level:	Cost:
Mild/Moderate	Mild/Moderate	$ - $$

RUNG 3: Lasers, Light System Treatments and Other Energy-based Treatments

EIGHT

8

THE LADDER
RUNG 3: LASERS, LIGHT SYSTEM TREATMENTS AND OTHER ENERGY-BASED TREATMENTS

Once you have your topical treatment plan all squared away, and you've explored if certain facials or peels are right for you, it could be the right time to begin thinking about laser or energy-based treatments for some additional anti-aging intervention. This rung offers the first level of intervention beyond topicals. Rung 3 features moderately expensive, relatively accessible treatment plans with **mild/moderate** benefit and risk.

Energy can be delivered in many ways to affect change. Energy delivery can be based in laser, light, radiofrequency, ultrasound or other means. Let's go through these individually here.

LASER is an acronym for *light amplification by stimulated emission of radiation*. This means high intensity light is used to target a specific area in the skin: pigment in hair, pigment in brown spots, hemoglobin in blood vessels or water in collagen. The heat is delivered to the target to affect the issue. In other words, the laser delivers heat to the skin in a controlled manner to destroy the target of the laser. Lasers can also be used for hair removal and tattoo removal. Lasers are mostly about maintenance and repair, but some physicians (including me) believe that the cell turnover you get with resurfacing lasers can be protective against some types of sun damage.

Lasers are typically the next rung on The Ladder if you fall in the 20-40 age range, and are starting to see signs of aging, scarring or discoloration that are not controlled or treated with topicals alone. With regularly scheduled laser treatments we can target signs of sun damage and resurface the skin for wrinkles, age spots, acne scarring, and texture irregularities. While recovery and side effects vary depending on the treatment you receive, all treatments improve the skin's condition and stimulate the skin's natural healing processes. Like any noninvasive treatment, lasers manipulate the skin and therefore have potential side effects. However, if you are receiving treatment from a qualified dermatologist, the risk of side effect will be minimal. There are a few different laser technologies available, and you and your dermatologist can decide which is the best option for you.

Laser Tattoo Removal – Laser tattoo removal has been around for decades now, but recent advances have allowed these lasers to become more effective for more colors. In the past we have really only been able to do a great job removing darker colors such as black, but new advancements have improved treatments for greens, yellows, reds and oranges. Laser tattoo removal targets the pigment that is deep in the skin with specific wavelengths based on the color of the tattoo pigment. Multiple treatments are required, but with advancements in technology, the number of treatments has also decreased from 15 treatments to now, 5-8. Side effects of laser tattoo removal include pigmentary alteration, scarring and even infection. The same safety precautions apply here as similar procedures. Make sure that if you are one of the rare people that has a side effect, there is a medical director on site who is able to see you for any problems or complications.

Laser For Red Spots and Blood Vessels - Laser for red spots and blood vessels targets the hemoglobin under the skin with a specific laser or light wavelengths. The heat is delivered to the hemoglobin causing destruction of the red spots or blood vessels. Multiple different lasers as well as light-based sources can be used to target hemoglobin and remove redness. The brand of laser is less important in this area than your practitioner's experience in treating blood vessels. Look at before and after pictures of your practitioner's work, ask how many years of experience with the laser they have, and find out why they chose the one that they did.

Laser For Brown Spots – Laser for brown spots is similar to laser for red spots and blood vessels, in that specific lasers or light sources can be used to target the brown spots. These target melanin in the skin. This pigment can be heated and brought to the surface where it will naturally slough off. Multiple different brands are available for this purpose also; but again, the brand is less important than your provider's experience with this light source and the results they can achieve with the laser that they work with.

Both lasers for red and brown have very little discomfort and very little downtime besides a small amount of blotchiness and swelling that resolves over a day or two. The brown areas can be brown for about a week before they fall off, and the discomfort with these lasers is minimal and feels like a rubber band snapping on your skin.

Laser Hair Reduction - Laser hair reduction (LHR) has come along way since the old days of extreme discomfort and 15 treatments. Advances in technology have allowed laser hair reduction to be a relatively painless procedure that can be performed in fewer treatments with great results. Personally, we use the light sheer device by Lumenis® in my office. This advanced technology has been the gold standard in laser hair reduction for at least a decade. Recent advancements including cooled tips and suction based devices have allowed for an almost completely painless experience, as well as being able to treat an entire leg in less than 15 minutes. You can still get great results with the older devices, but one of the reasons I never had laser hair removal prior to the new devices is that the discomfort was quite significant. The advanced technology has basically eliminated that problem. For more information about LHR, head to Chapter 12.

Laser Resurfacing – Laser resurfacing is used to treat wrinkles, acne scars, and texture irregularities. This used to be done in the operating room only with about 3 weeks of downtime, but advances in technology have allowed faster recovery and the ability to do it in the office while you are awake. There are many laser resurfacing brands out there but most are either CO_2 or erbium lasers, both are gases used to target water in the skin and direct heat to a specific layer. I tell my patients we can turn heat up or down depending on how much downtime they have and how intense a treatment we want.

Laser resurfacing can be either non-ablative or ablative (Ablative is more intense as the name suggests). Non-ablative laser resurfacing delivers heat to the deeper layers of the skin without doing a lot of damage to the very top layer of the skin. After the procedure patients are typically red with a sunburned look for 1-3 days and may have a mild sandpaper like peeling. Ablative resurfacing removes a percentage of the top layer of the skin to affect more superficial changes in addition to the collagen stimulation down deep. The ablative resurfacing has more scaling and peeling than non-ablative and takes 7-10 weeks to completely recover. As the skin heals a newer, tighter layer of skin forms. The full results can be expected 9-12 months after the procedure.

What Are Fractionated Lasers?

I have patients coming in all the time asking for fractionated lasers, sometimes by a brand that their friend has had, or they heard a radio ad about it. Fractionated lasers were invented to improve the downtime associated with laser resurfacing. About 20-30 years ago resurfacing had a higher risk of infection and scarring and took about 3 weeks to heal. Now with fractionated lasers we are able to provide great benefits without as much risk and downtime for patients. Fractionated lasers do not affect a full patch of skin. Instead they leave little islands of unaffected skin so the skin barrier's immune cells help heal the barrier laterally, rather than from below. You can also think of these islands like pixels in an image, where only some of the pixels are targeted in a single treatment.

There are many laser brands available out there currently and some more to come. Ask your dermatologist or plastic surgeon which one they have and why. You will be more satisfied with your treatment if you discuss laser treatment options with your doctor's office (someone you trust!) rather than looking for a treatment center that carries a specific brand.

Laser resurfacing increases collagen and improves fine lines, texture and irregularities. It also adds some tightening to the skin. Personally, I try and have a laser resurfacing treatment once per year.

Best Candidates For Laser Treatments
For the majority of laser treatments, ideal candidates have skin types 1, 2 or 3 and have mild to moderate signs of photoaging, scarring or discoloration. There are a couple reasons lighter-skinned people do better with laser treatments. The first is mechanic: the laser looks for pigment, and it has a more difficult time distinguishing between pigment of skin and pigment of the hair, spot or whatever else is being targeted.

The second is cultural: the advertising and cosmetic industry in United States has historically been more heavily weighted toward lighter skinned individuals, so the development of pigment correcting lasers reflects that. This has started to change, as we now commonly see women of color and different ethnicities endorsing products. We now have Kerry Washington and Eva Mendes endorsing popular skin care lines, and while there is a little bit of a shift, we still have a long way to go as the research has to catch up with our evolving culture. In the past 5 years there have been new treatments available that are safer for darker skin.

When my colleagues and I did the very first study of a fractional laser used on darker skin types in 2007, these lasers had been around a few years but had not yet been studied in darker skin types. We were looking to treat acne scarring, so we recruited people with skin Types 4, 5 and 6 who needed acne scarring treatment. They received free treatments in the study with full disclosure that the lasers might cause pigmentation. We were looking to find what percent were going to get pigmentation. Roughly 30 percent got pigmentation with the lasers, but all pigmentation had resolved in 6 months.

However, patients with darker skin are not exempt from laser or energy-based treatments. As I have mentioned before, *who* performs your treatments has a tremendous influence on the results and the potential for side effects. Choose a laser treatment professional with proper experience and qualifications for your specific needs and skin type. Part of getting optimal results also has to do with your own honesty. Be completely candid about your medical history, specifically what types of medications you have taken or are currently taking. You should also communicate whether you have had any problems with lasers or energy-based treatments in the past.

Light-Based Treatments (Photofacials)

Optimized Pulse Light, Intense Pulsed Light (IPL) and Broadband Light (BBL) are commonly called photofacials. These light-based treatments are not technically lasers, since lasers use a single wavelength to target water to destroy cells and stimulate collagen production. Instead, the photofacial uses low-level broadband light to deliver heat to the skin and stimulate collagen, minimize appearance of blood vessels (including rosacea) and improve the appearance of fine lines, wrinkles and other signs of sun damage.

LED-Based Acne Treatments

Having acne affects how you go about making cosmetic choices. This is where your dermatologist can be a great partner and advocate for helping you navigate your options. Home light treatments (which have recently become popular as a do-it-yourself treatment), can be heat-based, LED-based (red or blue light) or a combination of these. LED is an acronym for light emitting diode. You can get LEDs across the spectrum of light including visible, ultraviolet and infrared. Low level LED light therapy uses red and/or blue visible light. Blue light is used to disrupt the acne cycle, minimizing inflammation and killing bacteria, while red light is shown to improve collagen and wound healing. Depending on what you are looking for, both or one may be beneficial for you. [1] Some handheld devices deliver heat to the pimple, and that heat kills the bacteria that cause the pimples. Some devices use a combination of heat and LED. These devices range in price from $150-$300, but last quite a while so the investment may be worth it to you if you suffer from acne.

You can also use less expensive over-the-counter zit-zapping creams, which are typically salicylic acid or benzoyl peroxide-based. These are available in the acne aisle at your pharmacy. Your dermatologist or

Zit Zapper Devices

At-home zit treatment and complexion devices are gaining popularity, and they are also advancing quite a bit. The more expensive options are likely to have the most benefit, using low level blue and red light therapy to kill zit-causing bacteria, reduce inflammation and stimulate collagen. While I will be the first to say these at home devices are becoming more reliable, don't forget to do your research before adding one of these to your cart. Most of the at-home devices require daily or frequent use for an extended period of time before results can be realized. Keep your expectations realistic. For your own safety and health, over-the-counter devices do not have the strength or effectiveness of treatments provided by your dermatologist. Here are a few devices you may have seen and how they work.

- **no!no!® Skin** is a popular brand you may have seen on TV. The device delivers Light & Heat Energy (LHE®) technology to improve pimples.
- **Zeno Hot Spot** is the smallest of the zit zappers and it uses gentle heat to kill bacteria that causes acne. This brand has both a mini and a professional version.
- **Neutrogena® Light Therapy** uses red and blue light therapy, and helps reduce bacteria and inflammation in order to help minimize pimples.
- **Tria®** - This device claims to use the exact blue light intensity offered in professional treatments. The reviews are positive, though you have to purchase new cartridges every 300 minutes of use. If you're looking for a more intensive maintenance regimen this could be something to look into. Remember, there are many other devices and certainly more to come. If you have specific questions about them ask your dermatologist or experienced skin care professional.

primary care doctor can also write a prescription for a spot treatment, which are usually a topical benzoyl peroxide mixed with clindamycin or erythromycin.

Ultrasound Devices
Devices driven by ultrasound have been common for years and use safe ultrasound waves to administer to the deep layers of the skin in order to promote collagen formation and tightening. Ultrasound was once common for skin tightening, but advances in radiofrequency technology have lessened ultrasound's popularity in this space. There does seem to still be a lot of interest for a procedure call an "ultrasound facial," which is more or less an add-on offered by estheticians. This is relatively painless, as it does not penetrate into the deeper layers of the skin. If you are interested in doing this with your esthetician, understand that it is not as effective as your physician-based models that go deeper, but can provide some noticeable results. I'll briefly touch on ultrasound as it relates to skin tightening again in Rung 5: *Minimally Invasive Procedures: Tightening, Contouring and Lifting.*

Radiofrequency
Technology has advanced to include tightening options for both the face and body that do not involve ultrasound, light or laser. Radiofrequency has many medical and cosmetic uses. In cosmetic application, radiofrequency waves are used to deliver heat to the dermal tissue and stimulate collagen and elastin production. New technology now exists where radiofrequency is delivered deeper into the skin for significant tightening. I'll speak of this more in Rung 5.

Other Energy-based Treatments
In this section I've listed a few other treatments and devices you might come across in your research for what's right for you. If you are considering using any of the following, figure out what it is you want to treat and talk to your dermatologist to see what better options are available now.

Cosmetic Electrical Stimulation
Cosmetic electrical stimulation of the skin is a type of cosmetic treatment that uses low electrical currents to try to tighten and lift the skin. This can

be used on both the face and body. While this procedure was an important step for the advancement of noninvasive technology, as we would not have the great devices like FORMA Plus™, FaceTite™ and BodyTite™ without this initial invention, the results of deep radiofrequency, surgical facelifts and newer body contouring devices are now much more effective.

Microcurrent Electrical Neuromuscular Stimulation (MENS)

MENS is used to treat signs of aging and damage from sun exposure and scarring. MENS is applied to the surface of the skin and uses positively and negatively charged probes that deliver a very small, direct current to small organelles in the skin. These currents mimic the natural electrical currents within our bodies to encourage the body's natural regenerative processes. This stimulation is thought to tighten muscles by stimulating the release of ATP (*adenosine triphosphate*), which stimulates collagen and elastin as well as builds muscle. Most people do not feel any contraction with these. There is some evidence that collagen and elastin may be increased. There are more effective options if you are looking for collagen stimulation. None of my dermatologist friends use these, and they get the devices for free! That's saying something.

Galvanized Microcurrent

This is applied to the surface of the skin and is a constant current that cleanses the skin by breaking down hardened oils in pores (fittingly known as *desincrustation*) and applies a small direct current which helps nourishing substances penetrate into the tissues more easily. If you are trying to break down oils in the skin and allow medications such as antioxidants or peels to penetrate better, galvanized microcurrent could be the appropriate treatment for you. This can be done by an aesthetician as part of your facial.

Faradic Treatment

This is applied to the surface of the skin and firms and tones the facial tissue by repeatedly contracting the muscles with a short, direct electrical pulse. The treatment also increases muscle metabolism, which helps the muscle remove waste faster. Named after Michael Faraday, the faradic treatment is also called the *neuromuscular electrical stimulation* (NMES) and is safe to use for both face and body.

High Frequency Treatment

This uses a low-current, high-frequency wand on the surface of the skin to condition the skin and promote superficial healing and natural exfoliation. High-frequency treatment can also help minimize pores, mild puffiness and mild acne.

Do DIY Electrical Stimulation Devices Work?

If you are looking to an at-home electrical stimulation device, I recommend considering what you want the device to do, and then do some research as to whether this product is giving others the benefits it may be claiming on the packaging. At-home electrical current devices often list collagen stimulation as a main benefit a patient can enjoy. There is likely a small amount of collagen stimulation from the at-home (or spa) devices that use electrical current to try to induce collagen. In order to stimulate more collagen you must heat deeper layers of the skin, such as with physician-administered ultrasound or radiofrequency treatments.

Recovery, Risks and Precautions

While lasers and other energy-based treatments typically don't require much down time, you will have a mild pink color to your skin and mild swelling for about two days. More aggressive resurfacing treatments can take anywhere between 1-2 weeks for full recovery. During this time, you can expect your skin to recover and you will need to follow the post care instructions given to you by your doctor to promote the best healing.

Risks for energy-based treatments are generally low with proper pre- and post-procedure care. Risks include infection, scarring and pigmentation problems, most of which can almost always be prevented with proper operation from a skilled professional. Discuss your skin type and any precautions that should be taken that are specific to you and your medical history.

Although you can have laser resurfacing done at any time of year, I typically recommend my patients receive treatments in the fall, winter or early spring, and there is less threat of sun exposure during recovery. Sun exposure not only undoes some of the benefits of the laser making (it is less bang for your buck), but there are also other pigmentation risks if you have significant exposure after laser. If you spend most of your time indoors, you have more flexibility on timing than a skier or baseball player.

Going Further - Combination Treatments

As people's lives get busier and maximizing downtime and effectiveness becomes more and important, combination treatments have increased popularity. In our office we offer multiple different combination treatments for our patients. One of our popular noninvasive combinations treatments is called the ThreeForMe™.Using Intense Pulsed Light (IPL) technology with the ICON resurfacing laser, the procedures target three problems at once—sun damage and brown spots, wrinkles and facial veins. This procedure is a combined treatment for clients seeking to improve the visible effects of sun exposure with one treatment. The treatment first addresses brown and red skin discoloration with specific tailored settings for your skin type. Then wrinkles and collagen are treated with an erbium-fractionated laser designed to stimulate collagen and elastin production.

While there is some mild discomfort similar to the snapping of a rubber band against the skin during the procedure and a warming feeling afterward, most patients tolerate the combination procedure very well. After the treatment, you'll notice improvement in the facial veins and brown spots within a week. The collagen stimulation continues for 6 months after your treatment so the fine lines and wrinkles of your face will show more improvement each day. Many great dermatologists that I know offer this or something similar for their patients to help treat the many areas of sun damage all at once.

Risk–Benefit–Cost

Risk Level:	Benefit Level:	Cost:
Mild/Moderate	Mild/Moderate	$$

RUNG 4: Injectables

NINE

9

THE LADDER
RUNG 4: INJECTABLES

The fourth rung of The Ladder hosts neuromodulators (BOTOX®, Dysport® and Xeomin®) and dermal fillers (Juvéderm® ®, Restylane® and Radiesse®). This rung offers a level of treatment somewhat parallel to Rung 3 in terms of cost and risk factor. It must be performed by a licensed, board-certified physician in many states, and a certified nurse, nurse practitioner or physician assistant in others. Rung 4 features moderately expensive, relatively accessible treatment plans with **moderate** benefit and risk.

While both neuromodulators and dermal fillers work to minimize fine lines and wrinkles, they are working on the tissues in very different ways. A simple way to remember the difference is Neuromodulators *relax* and fillers *replenish*. Neuromodulators offer short-term benefits while dermal fillers can last 6-24 months. Injectable procedures can take anywhere between 15-45 minutes.

Neuromodulators
Next to facelifts and liposuction, neuromodulators are one of the defining procedures of cosmetic medicine. Neuromodulators are made from botulinum toxin Type A, or the same bacteria that causes botulism. This bacteria was discovered in World War II era but was only first approved by the FDA in 2002 for reducing facial wrinkles. It works by inhibiting communication in the nerves in the injected tissue to reduce the appearance of fine lines and wrinkles. In other words, it's a muscle relaxer that lasts about 4 months. The most famous neuromodulator brand is, of

course, Botox®, while other big brands include Dysport® and Xeomin®. Neuromodulators are used primarily in the upper third of the face where expression lines form. The repetitive motions and loss of collagen cause expression lines over time. Neuromodulators are typically used for forehead wrinkles, crow's feet, brow "lifting," frown lines and marionette lines, bunny lines and upper lips.

Neuromodulators can also be used to reduce excess sweating. This is commonly done for sweaty foreheads and armpits, but also for hands. I have had patients who wear gloves all day for their professions and deal with sweaty hands. One of my patients even develops pools of sweat in the bottom of her gloves, which puts a real damper on her workday (Of course that pun was intended). To manage her hand sweating, she has injections of botulinum toxin Type A into her palms and fingers. Neuromodulator injections dramatically improve her quality of life at work and allow her to manage the problem.

BOTOX® and Dysport® are particularly useful for forehead wrinkles, but can be used to reduce the appearance of crow's feet, lip lines and neck bands as well. These injectables tend to work best when used continuously because they slow the progression of wrinkles over time.

Note: When talking about neuromodulators, I say the word "injectable" with caution since it will be no time before many of these treatments will be available in topical form.

Dermal Fillers
Dermal Fillers, soft fillers or "injectable implants" according to the FDA, temporarily improve deeper lines and restore volume. Fillers replenish smoothness and fullness to the face. Fillers can be used to treat deep creases in the nasolabial folds, depressions in the temples, cheeks and under the eyes, and smoothing out acne scars. Filler is not approved for breast or buttocks augmentation, and while it is FDA approved for the top of the hands, but it is not approved for the feet.

Unlike neuromodulators, dermal fillers plump up and fill the depressed areas. Fillers are considered a non-surgical rejuvenation treatment. While dermal fillers are advancing in effectiveness, it takes a lot of filler to get the "liquid facelift" as they are called online. We will talk about facelifts in length in Rung 6, but the short of the matter is this: facelifts are at the top of The Ladder for a reason. They are the most effective. However, it is true that many people do not need that drastic of a lift, and filler is just the amount of "lift" they need.

Dermal fillers can be categorized as either natural or synthetic. Natural fillers are mainly composed of hyaluronic acid, while synthetic fillers contain collagen stimulators like poly-L-lactic acid or calcium. Most fillers available in the U.S. are hyaluronic acid based including those in the Juvéderm® and Restylane® family. Most fillers are absorbed by the body in 6 months to 2 years and are called biodegradable. The only filler that is not absorbed and is currently FDA approved is PMMA, a semi-permanent filler. This type of filler is approved for correcting acne scars and the nasolabial folds.

When choosing the right filler for you, there are a few factors to consider. First, how much help do you need? The patient with minimal fine lines will not necessarily be receiving the same type of filler as the patient with deep-set wrinkles or hollowed temples. Consider the way the skin ages and recall the skin as a multi-layered structure. You have your structural support provided by the cheekbones, you have the muscle layer contributing to the dynamic expressions of the face, and you have the fat pads and skin contributing to volume. There is a laundry list of fillers to reflect the range of goals a patient can have. We want to think about the different types of fillers by ingredient or by brand. Many brands have several products that vary in thickness, longevity and placement areas, and can help you achieve different goals. You have probably seen brands like Juvéderm®. Well, Juvéderm® now has five different types of filler to choose from. It is important for you and your provider to sit down and figure out which of these is best for you and in what area you want treated. Do not purchase fillers online, as these products are likely to be unapproved or counterfeit products. It is not safe to use these products at home.

Hyaluronic Acid Fillers
Hyaluronic acid fillers, such as Restylane®, Volbella®, Belotero®, Voluma®

and Juvéderm®, are considered natural fillers and are biodegradable. They are ideal for first time filler patients because the results are consistently positive with little side effects. Hyaluronic acid fillers have a much lower chance of causing a reaction, since hyaluronic acid is a natural constituent of our skin. However no treatment is risk-free, since people can have allergic reactions to anything including the small amount of lidocaine in the filler tube. The results from hyaluronic acid fillers can last anywhere between 6 months to 2 years depending on location placed and product chosen.

Hyaluronic acid fillers can be thought of in three general categories based on consistency. When I explain this in my office to patients I let them know that in general, hyaluronic acid fillers come in thin, medium and thick.

- The thin products are used in thinner skin such as around the eyes and mouth. You can think of this type as more of a fine line eraser. This is also commonly used to smooth fine lines, lip lines or plump the lips.
- The medium products are for medium folds such as nasolabial folds and marionette lines.
- The thicker products can be used for deeper placement on cheekbones or in the temple region to elevate tissue.

There are new variations on hyaluronic acid fillers all the time, so it is best to get a plan customized for your specific anatomy. For example, there are some patients who have thicker, oily skin and can tolerate thicker products better than people who have thinner, dry skin. Hyaluronic acid fillers can last 6-12 months in the lip, 12-18 months for the marionettes, and nasolabial folds and up to 2 years for the cheeks and temples.

Here is a list of the most common hyaluronic acid fillers approved in the U.S. (Please not that may more are available in Europe that are not approved state-side).

- **Juvéderm® Ultra** is a thinner product which can help to augment the lips or help with smaller fine lines around the mouth.

- **Juvéderm® Ultra Plus** is a medium-thickness injectable restore the volume and the youthful contours of your face around the mouth, nose and forehead. Juvéderm is also commonly used under the eyes and for acne scars.

- **Vollure®** is of medium thickness, is FDA approved and is designed to help correct nasolabial folds and marionette lines.

- **Volbella®** is a hyaluronic acid dermal filler that augments the lips and improves wrinkles and fine lines around the mouth. Volbella® is ideal for treating the most delicate areas of the face and has applications for thin skin areas such as the tear troughs, but only in experienced hands.

- **Voluma®** is formulated to treat age-related, midface volume loss, including the cheekbone area. It lifts the skin and gives not only volume improvement, but used correctly a lift to the face. Voluma® is approved by the FDA to be effective for up to 2 years.

- **Restylane®** is an HA filler made and FDA approved for volume restoration and improvement in lines. There are five types of Restylane® currently: Silk, Lyft, Refyne, Defyne and the standard Restylane®. Silk is used primarily to restore volume to the lips and surrounding lines. Lyft is used primarily for the cheek and Refyne and Defyne around the mouth and nasolabial folds. The standard Restylane is also used for fine lines and nasolabial folds. Restylane products last 6-12 months depending on the area treated and product placement.

- **Belotero** is another HA filler used primarily for fine lines and volume restoration. It also lasts 6-12 months depending on area and placement.

Calcium hydroxylapatite (Radiesse®)

Most commonly known by the brand Radiesse®, calcium hydroxylapatite is biodegradable and synthetic. It is a unique filler made of calcium hydroxyapatite. It is FDA approved to treat areas of the face as well as rejuvenation of the hands. Currently I use this mostly for hand rejuvenation as well as facial rejuvenation in the nasolabial folds and marionette lines. It does a great job. I tell my patients that this filler reliably holds for 12 months and may in some people last 18 months.

Poly-L-lactic Acid Fillers

Poly-L-lactic acid fillers (PLLA) are a type of synthetic filler that are biodegradable according to the FDA. This filler has been called permanent by some sources, but the FDA lists it as "lasting 2 years." In my experience this filler lasts longer than 2 years but does eventually reabsorb. PLLA is considered a "stimulant" because it is collagen stimulating. You will not see immediate results with this filler because it calls on the body's natural collagen production systems. Rather, optimal results will appear after 6 weeks and 3-5 treatments. This filler is used to treat deep wrinkles, improve volume loss in the midface area, including the cheeks; and fill nasolabial folds and marionettes. One of the most common Poly-L-lactic Acid filler brand is Sculptra®

Synthetic Fillers

Synthetic fillers have their own positive attributes. They tend to last longer than the natural fillers and they can stimulate your body to make more of its own collagen once they are placed. But, reactions to synthetic fillers are more severe because they are products that are not normally in the body and are more difficult to manage. As they last longer and cannot be dissolved easily, any problems you may experience will be harder to treat. The hyaluronic acid fillers can be dissolved with an enzyme called hyaluronidase, though there is really no such enzyme for the synthetics.

Polymethylmethacrylate (PMMA)

PMMA is another type of non-biodegradable, synthetic filler that lasts over a year according to the FDA. It is generally used when a patient is looking for a more permanent filler option, and in my experience it lasts longer than 2 years. The filler sits beneath the skin in microspheres and adds support and volume to the skin. The FDA-approved brand for this type of filler is Bellafill® which is approved for volume restoration in the nasolabial folds and marionettes as well as to treat acne scars. Bellafill® is suspended in bovine collagen (cow) and does require a test spot before treatment to make sure you are not allergic to the product. It is a good choice for specific patients.

Fat Injections

How exciting that plastic surgery now allows us to fulfill our wishes to take some fat from "here" and move it to "there." Although technically not a "filler" most of the time fat injections can be used in a similar way to filler so they are worth mentioning here. Facial rejuvenation using fat grafting or fat injection is the process by which a plastic surgeon uses your own fat cells, harvested from fat deposits on your lower body for instance, to create a smoother, fuller, more youthful shape to your lips, nose, eyes, jowls, temples or cheeks. Usually fat can do most everything that filler can do. It's also your own tissue, so there is no risk for allergy and it is rich in growth factors.

So now for the catch. Fat has to be harvested from your body with liposuction in order to process and use it for volume restoration. This liposuction is considered a surgical procedure and has its own risks associated. I commonly use fat for my patients that are having another type of surgery and need some volume in their face. I also use it for those who cannot use other fillers for any reason, or for people who only want to use their own tissue. In our office we have tailored this procedure so it can be done in the office with local numbing medication for both the liposuction area and the area the fat will be placed. We do this to make it available to those people that are not having surgery. I have to say this is the only time that I have been able to say, "I love fat." With fat comes the growth factors and other stimulators that your body naturally makes, so it is a win-win. Your dermatologist and plastic surgeon can help you decide which products are best for you.

Fat Injections

People ask me if I prefer fat. I say, "Every day of the week and twice on Sunday!" Although, it is more involved than filler.

GOING FURTHER

Combination Treatments: Neuromodulators and Dermal Fillers
Since dermal filler and neuromodulators are only FDA approved for certain areas of the soft tissue, it is common for your doctor to advise a combination approach to treating signs of aging. In this plan of treatment, the patient receives dermal fillers and neuromodulator injections for optimal results. Despite having a slightly longer appointment, there is no known additional risks for combining these procedures.

Neuromodulators for Prevention
While Xeomin® Botox® and Dysport® were originally created to target moderate to severe frown lines between the eyebrows, I am seeing younger and younger patients asking for neuromodulators just as the lines start to etch so they can be prevented. If you have room in your budget to used neuromodulators as a preventative measure, I say go for it. However I wouldn't consider it essential.

My mother and I have very similar anatomy, which makes for a great example of this. My mom had not received any injections and had etched the lines on her brow fairly deeply prior to me becoming a dermatologist (and prior to BOTOX® being invented). While I now give her some treatment for them, it will take a long time for her body to fill those lines in all the way if ever. In contrast, I started using neuromodulators in my 30s preventively, right when I started to see those lines on my forehead. I literally have not etched a line, even though I have the same anatomy as my mom has. I have kept up my BOTOX® and have been able to prevent them from forming.

Once the line is etched to the lionene stage (or etching that give us that similar look of a lion), it's more difficult to use these products as preventative because this treatment does not *reverse* signs of aging. It halts communication that would otherwise pronounce them. While it's a little bit more difficult to make drastic cellular change using neuromodulators, you can certainly improve the appearance of lines as a maintenance measure, even once they have formed. One of my patients had deep furrows between her brows and she wanted them gone. We discussed it would take one treatment every 3 months for a few years. She kept it up and after two years they were gone, but it took time as they had been etched for 40 years.

Microcurrent or Botox: Which Is Best For You?

I have seen this come up a few times, which is perplexing as one inhibits muscle contraction and the other amplifies it (in theory). While neuromodulators like BOTOX® inhibit muscle and keep it from etching lines, microcurrent treatments help the body release ATP and stimulate muscles. If I was to make an argument for microcurrent, it would be that it is possible that current delivers heat to the skin and stimulates some collagen; but microcurrent and neuromodulators are not in the same class. If you love microcurrent technology, you can use it. Just know that I consider microcurrent as a way to help keep the skin in good condition *before* you need BOTOX® and fillers. Think of microcurrent treatments like facials and peels. They are supplementary treatments on the path to a more youthful appearance prior to reaching the higher rungs of The Ladder.

Risks and Precautions

While there is virtually no downtime for neuromodulators or dermal fillers, it is completely normal to experience mild redness, and swelling at the injection sites as well as temporary bruising. Using makeup to cover up those side effects should do the trick.

I advise first-time patients for injectables to begin with a small area for neuromodulators and one syringe of a temporary filler so we can assess the results and individual and decide how to proceed.

Despite the overwhelming demand for injectables, I find there are still a lot of questions about the possible negative effects of neurotoxins, like Botox®, on the body. For one, there are concerns whether the neurotoxin travels from the injection site to other parts of the body. Although this is a science-backed concern, as systemic botulism is a serious illness, there has not been a case of cosmetic doses of neurotoxin that cause systemic effects in the body that I am aware of. Neurotoxins have been available for cosmetic uses in the U.S. for over a decade and there are literally hundreds of thousands of injections done annually.

For filler, the possible complications are more real and I strongly advise people to never have this procedure done in a location that does not take it seriously. As with any product being placed under the skin, infection is possible. Your provider should be wearing clean gloves that have not touched other areas, and will clean the skin with a broad-spectrum cleanser to rid the skin of as much bacteria and other pathogens as possible.

In terms of placement, fillers can occasionally result in some lumpiness around the injection site, though this is usually temporary. If the product is injected too superficially, the patient may experience a nodule underneath the skin or a bluish tint, which is also temporary. Patients may also be able to feel the filler beneath your skin, but these effects will go away over time. If any of these usually temporary side effects remain longer than desired, most can be dissolved by your physician.

While it is very rare, filler can get into a blood vessel in the face, an emergency that requires hyaluronidase (the enzyme that dissolves most filler) and other modalities right away. Your provider should have hyaluronidase on hand to dissolve the filler immediately if any problems arise. Hyaluronidase is expensive, only the most knowledgeable and experienced providers will have it on hand. Only use an injector that has this available. Ask for it, and if they do not have it, it's in your best interest to leave.

Risk-Benefit-Cost

Risk Level:	Benefit Level:	Cost:
Moderate	Moderate	$$$

RUNG 5: Tightening, Contouring and Lifting Procedures

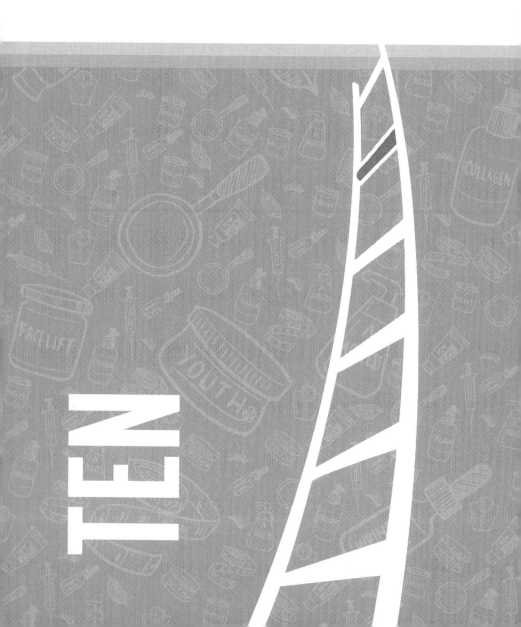

TEN

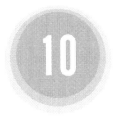

THE LADDER
RUNG 5: TIGHTENING, CONTOURING AND LIFTING PROCEDURES

One step up from dermal fillers and neuromodulators you will find noninvasive (or minimally invasive) contouring, tightening and lifting treatments. Rung 5 demonstrates the continuously advancing field of noninvasive options for fat reduction, facial and neck tightening, skin tightening and smoothing procedures.

Despite these advancements, qualified, licensed physicians must always perform or supervise these procedures. These treatments do give great results for areas that 10 years ago could only be treated surgically, though they are not as involved as surgical procedures. Rung 5 features more expensive treatment plans with **moderate/high** benefit and risk.

Since procedures on this rung are not as involved as surgical procedures, it is no surprise they are growing in popularity. Skin tightening and fat reduction procedures have increased by at least five percent each year since 2015 when some of the first noninvasive treatments became available.

In 2017 cellulite treatments increased by 19 percent in one year. Tightening, lifting and contouring treatments like CoolSculpting® and Kybella® also saw a 7 percent and 12 percent increase respectively.

When you think of noninvasive tightening and contouring procedures, you may also think of certain advertisements you may have seen that claim they can be completed during a lunch break. Ads are great at piquing patient interest, but they leave many questions unanswered. Be cautious of such informal offerings and be sure to speak with a plastic surgeon or dermatologist who individualizes your care for what is best for your situations and treats you like a person first, not just another procedure.

While these procedures are organized between the noninvasive and the minimally invasive, they are all still *procedures*. Noninvasive procedures (or ones that do not puncture the skin) have less risk and less downtime, but risk still exists. Minimally invasive procedures are only getting more and more effective, sometimes producing results close to surgical procedures. The minimally invasive procedures still come with potential risks and should always be performed under the supervision of a physician. Before you say "yes" to a minimally invasive procedure, ask yourself: *Do I understand the risks? Can I consent to this procedure and adhere to post procedure instructions? Who will take care of me if I have one of the uncommon side effects?*

The last question here may be the most important one. If there will not be a physician available or supervising if you need prescription, have an infection, or are in pain, then receive treatment somewhere else.

Not all injectors, laser providers, or noninvasive options are created equal, so be sure they are well qualified to perform that procedure (and well qualified to perform any necessary corrections). We will talk more about finding a qualified professional for a procedure in Chapter 13.

Non- and Minimally Invasive Fat Reduction and Contouring Therapies
Our relationship with fat is a complicated one. While we've recently accepted "good" fat back into our diets, we still have a hard time accepting there's good fat we carry in our body too. The reason for this is twofold. First, we typically associate fat with *unwanted* or stubborn fat pockets that keep us from having a proportional figure. But fat actually has several purposes and is stored in different ways. Our bodies house fat in two areas: subcutaneous or "pinchable" fat, and visceral or intra-abdominal fat. Visceral fat surrounds and protects vital organs beneath the muscle layer, while subcutaneous fat sits above the muscle, just below the skin. Visceral fat is comparatively more dangerous to the body (if it's in excess amounts) and is associated with increase risk of heart disease. Unfortunately, this

type of fat cannot be removed surgically and can also be hereditary. Visceral fat can only be decreased with healthy diet and exercise. Surgery and noninvasive fat reduction procedures allow us to remove subcutaneous fat.

Subcutaneous fat, in healthy amounts, serves a function in the body. This type of fat insulates and cushions our bones, blood vessels and skin, protecting us from bruising. It also provides energy. This fat can also be removed through various fat reduction therapies or used for grafting.

Even the slimmest of us come across mid-life widening, or the accumulation of body fat around the middle section as we enter our 40s and 50s. Fat just becomes a little more stubborn. As women, we lose our estrogens, lose the hourglass figure and develop the apple shape. For men, their testosterone levels decrease, which can lead to unwanted soft or pudgy areas where they used to be toned. That's where body sculpting comes in. The ideal candidates for noninvasive or minimally invasive fat reduction is looking for contouring changes, not weight loss. Because the noninvasive procedures rely on the body to metabolize and get rid of the fat on its own, fat reduction or sculpting procedures take a few treatments and a few months to get your ideal outcome.

One of the biggest questions we get about fat-reduction therapies is whether the procedure is permanent. The answer is *yes,* the fat cells that are destroyed with the treatment do not come back, but the caveat is you can still gain weight again by increasing the size of the fat cells you have left. If you control your weight afterward the results are permanent. After these sculpting procedures you will notice your clothes fit better and you may even be able to go down a size.

Fat Freezing (Cryolipolysis)

Fat freezing has an interesting invention story. Dermatology has long known about the phenomenon called *Popsicle Panniculitis*, which caused dents in the cheeks when children held popsicles in the same spot for too long. This left children with dimples and Harvard researchers with a novel idea for fat-reduction therapy. Fast forward a few years and you'll find that the idea of cold targeting fat cells has gone mainstream with the advent of

My Favorite Thing About The 'F' Word

As we age, fat becomes instrumental in maintaining our youthful appearance. If you think about the fat pads beneath our skin, the more fat you have, the more volume you have in the face. Have you ever noticed how people with a little extra weight look younger? Despite our tendency to fight fat-accumulation as we age, having the right fat actually plays in our favor. Heavier people don't lose as much volume in their face, causing them to look younger for longer. By no means am I saying to go out and gain 20 pounds. That could actually have some pretty negative health effects in other departments. If you refer to my explanation of the aging face and body, you will recall volume loss is only a fraction of the ways we age.

CoolSculpting®. Who could have imagined that something like *popsicles* would be the key to unlocking a revolutionary new way to shed fat?

CoolSculpting® is now the fastest growing fat dissolving device in the country. The procedure contours the body in areas where stubborn, fat pockets reside. Some of the more popular areas include the bulges around the bra area, the abdomen and flanks, as well as the inner and outer thighs. With the addition of DualSculpting (the process of using two CoolSculpting® machines at the same time), and the new, fast applicators—treatment times are fairly short (about 30-60 minutes) and the results are only getting better. In my opinion, this procedure is one of the best noninvasive fat reduction treatments on the market.

Heat Therapy For Fat Reduction

Another noninvasive option actually melts the fat over time. SculpSure® is an FDA-approved technology that uses lasers to heat fat cells without damaging the skin's surface. Like CoolSculpting®, your body processes the fat cells and eliminates them through natural cell elimination processes. Patients begin to see results over the next 3 months and as soon as 6 weeks. During the 25-minute session, you will feel a cooling sensation, which helps to soothe the skin under the intense heat. Because the procedure is noninvasive, you are able to carry on with your day like normal afterward.

Other Fat-Reduction Technology

Unlike fat freezing, products like Liposonix® and Vanquish™ use heat technology to target the superficial layer of fat. These types of fat-reduction therapy products do not require any downtime and are less involved than SculpSure® or CoolSculpting®. The energy waves disrupt the fat cells, causing them to break down, which the body can then metabolize. The heat from the energy also stimulates some collagen production. The treatment usually takes about 30 minutes, though anywhere between 5-10 sessions are recommended for maximum results. You are a good candidate for this procedure if your physician can pinch an inch of fat around the midsection. Since these procedures are more superficial, they are generally less effective than the above mentioned cool or heat therapies.

Fat Dissolving (Kybella®)

The submental fat pocket located under the chin (better known as the *double-chin*) is an annoyance for both men and women, and it is unfortunately stubborn even when we are at our ideal weight. As a non-surgical alternative to liposuction or neck lift, fat-dissolving injections like Kybella® can be a safe alternative. Kybella® is composed of the same material found in the gallbladder that digests fat in your G.I. tract. When injected under the skin into the fat pocket of the chin, Kybella® destroys fat cells, causing the fat pocket to shrink. The injections are placed about 1 centimeter apart, and the number of injections needed is based on the size of the fat pocket, as well as the patient's desired results. This treatment is very effective and requires about 3-5 sessions for maximum results.

While Kybella® can result in some skin tightening, it is not approved by the FDA for treating skin sagging around the neck, commonly known as *turkey neck*.

TIGHTENING

Ultrasound for Skin Tightening

Again, ultrasound technology has been available for years for skin tightening. Recent advancements have made it more effective and comfortable. As technology advances to radiofrequency (explained over the next few sections) these devices are becoming less popular, but they remain a science-based option for tightening of the skin on the face, neck and chest to treat signs of aging. The most common and widely available option is called Ultherapy®. The result of this treatment is a subtle lift and tightening in the face. The results last for about one year and you will typically see the most results after months, as collagen needs time to produce. While there is no downtime, patients can expect mild discomfort during the procedure and mild redness and swelling afterward.

Radiofrequency for Tightening
For years patients have been looking for a non-surgical option for tightening and I have had a hard time recommending what has been previously available based on the cost to benefit ratio, until now. FaceTite™ and BodyTite™ offer minimally invasive tightening options that really work for the face/neck and body, respectively, while FORMA Plus™ offers a completely *noninvasive* option for no downtime.

BodyTite™ and FaceTite™ radiofrequency devices administer heat above and below the skin, sandwiching the skin between two probes. This is very effective and allows for more tightening then any device previously. The wand is passed under the skin by a board certified plastic surgeon delivering radiofrequency to the full thickness of the skin and tightening it up to 35 percent. These devices are available for body and face and have drastically improved what we can do without surgery. This procedure is as "scarless" as they come for minimally invasive options, requiring only small pore-sized ports for entry, and can be done in the office or the operating room depending on your specific needs.

FORMA Plus™ , on the other hand, is the new gold standard for skin tightening. It is noninvasive and less painful than other noninvasive options that have been around for a while. FORMA Plus™ rejuvenates and tightens the skin by heating heats the subdermal layers to promote collagen and tighten skin.

Radiofrequency with Assisted Lipoplasty

Radiofrequency treatments like BodyTite™ and FaceTite™ can also be performed with liposuction or lipoplasty. When performed with lipoplasty you can achieve tightening *and* contouring. This can also be performed in the office or in the operating room and a small port site the size of a spaghetti noodle is placed to insert the device. The device is moved over the area to be treated, using the heat technology to melt fat to be sucked away with liposuction, tighten skin and contour your body. This procedure is ideal for patients looking to firm and contour the face, jawline, stomach, arms, chest, knees or thighs.

Risk-Benefit-Cost

Risk Level:	Benefit Level:	Cost:
Moderate/High	Moderate/High	$$$-$$$$

Risks and Precautions

Although noninvasive and minimally invasive procedures have less risk than surgical procedures, because the skin and underlying tissues are manipulated or removed, there will always be risks. These risks can be mitigated when you receive treatment from a board-certified dermatologist or plastic surgeon's office. Before undergoing any of the procedures listed above, please review Chapter 13: *Choosing The Right Dermatologist or Plastic Surgeon.*

RUNG 6: Surgical Procedures

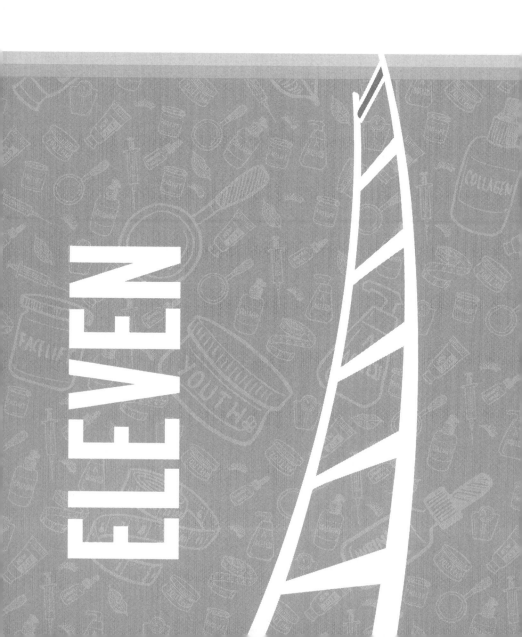

ELEVEN

THE LADDER
RUNG 6: SURGICAL PROCEDURES

The sixth and final rung is saved for surgical procedures. Rung 6 features more costly treatment plans with **high benefit** and the highest risk, relative to other treatments on The Ladder.

Surgery quite literally goes where noninvasive procedures can't, making long-term changes deep in the tissue to turn back your clock or enhance nearly any feature of the body. The most common surgical procedures since 2000 have been breast augmentation, eyelid surgery, facelift, liposuction and nose reshaping surgery. [1] Despite long-told stories of drastic, unnatural results from surgery (I am sure you can think of some celebrities without me naming any names), most patients are looking for subtle lifts, tucks and manageable reductions. The number of cosmetic surgeries performed in this country proves that each of us knows a handful of people that have had cosmetic surgery. Those are the ones we are talking about, the ones that look better, more refreshed, not overdone. With the advancement of noninvasive technology, there is some shift from surgical procedures to noninvasive procedures. While there are some procedures that must be performed surgically, noninvasive procedures can sometimes be performed first to "wait" on surgical ones, taking more of a stepladder approach. While you can dramatically improve the appearance of wrinkles around the nasolabial folds with injectables, for example, the best and most long-lasting results for deep wrinkles is still the facelift.

While surgical procedures have certainly improved the lives of countless patients, they are not for everyone. Surgical procedures sit at the top of

The Ladder because they are the most expensive procedures available and, because surgery is surgery, it poses some risks even to the healthiest patient. Most of these risks are manageable when you and your doctor have good communication and clear, shared expectations of your surgery from beginning to end.

On the flipside, it seems many patients do not perceive cosmetic surgery as having the same risks as a medical procedure, like heart surgery, for example. It is true that a person that needs heart surgery is, by definition, sick and at a greater risk than a healthy person, but surgery is still surgery. Though we only perform cosmetic elective surgeries on healthy patients, they should be treated with the same seriousness as medical procedures. Surgical procedures should always be performed in a licensed surgical facility that is accredited by your state, and your cosmetic surgery should be performed by a board-certified, experienced plastic surgeon. No matter what you are deciding to have done or how confident you may be about the procedure, it's important to plan your surgical procedure extensively with a plastic surgeon beforehand. These procedures are big, often exciting decisions, but they also come with some risk and should be treated with the time and planning they warrant. I can't say it enough, and I don't mind sounding like a broken record. Be your own best advocate (I'll likely say this again before the end of this book).

When Should You Have Surgery?
Deciding to have surgery is a big (and exciting) conversation with your doctor. While some patients would rather head to surgery immediately, others prefer to try less involved procedures first and work their way up from there. Your treatment plan will depend on your doctor's recommendations, the area you want to improve and your personal choice. We want to give you as much information as possible, without being too overwhelming, so you can feel informed about your decisions.

Whether you have come to a point where noninvasive procedures no longer help you achieve your goals, or you've been waiting for the proper moment to schedule your procedure, there are some questions worth asking yourself well before operation day.

1. Am I with a board-certified plastic surgeon?
2. Am I at an accredited surgery center?
3. Do I have reasonable expectations?
4. Have I met with my surgeon and feel comfortable with the plan?
5. Do I have all of my questions asked and answered?
6. Do I have my post-operative instructions?
7. Do I have someone to help me after surgery?

Let's talk about question three for a minute. Surgery can lead to some impressive results, however the idea is to enhance your natural aesthetic. I'm sure at some point you've taken a photo of your favorite celebrity hairstyle to your salon appointment. If your stylist has your best interests in mind, he or she will tell you honestly whether or not that style will suit your features—like when my stylist told me the haircut I wanted would look like I had a haystack on my head. I appreciated that. In this way, the expectations you have going into surgery should be realistic and fit your body.

A small percentage of patients see Dr. Timothy Janiga after a disappointed result from another surgeon or location. We want to reduce that chance as much as we can by starting off on the same page. No matter what procedure you have planned, you and your surgeon should be on the same page. Dr. Timothy Janiga's happiest patients went in with an accurate expectation for altering a feature to normalize it. So if you are getting a breast reduction for comfort, a breast augmentation to feel more feminine or a tummy tuck to correct some of the changes you experienced after having children, then your surgery can likely reach your expectations. Be honest with your surgeon about what you are trying to achieve. This way they can help guide these expectations.

How is your overall health?
Surgery is at the top of The Ladder, so before jumping to the top for a fat reduction procedure, we strongly advise that you have made necessary lifestyle changes (more vegetables, more cardio!).

If you're a smoker, surgery may not be possible until you quit. It's nothing personal, but nicotine actually shrinks your blood vessels, which can result in some complications. Many people seek to get a second opinion about this, and that's fine. For your safety, it is best to quit smoking at least 4-6 week before surgery.

Are you at a stable weight?
Before going undergoing surgery you should be at a stable weight (breast size too!) for at least a year. The logic behind this is simple: if your body is changing for whatever reason, it may continue to change after surgery and you may not be satisfied long term.

Overall you might be ready for surgery if you have realistic expectations, you are doing this for you and only you, and you are in a proper mental and physical state.
Surgery can typically be categorized in to three types:

Type 1- Face and neck
Type 2 - Breast
Type 3 - Body

Surgical Procedures: Type 1 - Face and Neck Procedures
Social media and selfies have a significant impact on our current culture. It's evident in the filters and editing tricks people and companies use on social media and in print to enhance people's looks. It is also evident in the recent uptick in facelift and neck lift requests. Facelift popularity dropped a bit in 2015, but just a year later numbers shot back up to one of the top five plastic surgery procedures in the United States. [2]

The most common surgical procedures for the face and neck are lifts and fat grafting. A facelift is a form of plastic surgery that serves to lift the skin and underlying structures of the face and neck. For decades, the surgical facelift has utilized superficial and deep tightening but with time even surgical facelifts have evolved. Modern facelifts may include fat grafting to restore underlying volume loss in those that need it at the same time. Fat grafting is the process of taking fat from somewhere else on the body—whether it's the tummy, thighs or the flank—and injecting it into the volume deficient area. This is particularly useful for women that are thin or have that hollowed look as they age. Unlike BOTOX® or a filler that wears off over time, a facelift is a physical removal of skin and tightening of underlying structures. Together, fat grafting and a facelift can improve signs of aging by 7-10 years in most people and some may get a 15-year boost.

How much does a face/neck lift cost?

This is a common question that does not have a firm answer, as each patient is different and each geographical area is different. A facelift in New York City is easily double what one in Michigan might be. Location of your procedure also matters. Some of the mini lifts can be performed in the office, which lowers the price, but not everyone is a candidate for the mini facelift. If you are going to the operating room you should plan to spend at a minimum $15,000 and up to $40,000 for a facelift. If you are a candidate for some of the in-office or mini procedures you can plan a minimum of $8,000 and up to $20,000. Remember that you may need add on procedures such as an eyelid lift that will add to the cost, which is why it is best to meet with a board-certified plastic surgeon in your area and get a specific quote based on what you want and need.

There are two main types of facelifts: the deep-plane (or traditional) facelift and SMAS facelift. All SMAS facelifts involve manipulation of the SMAS layer. The SMAS is the superficial muscular aponeurotic system, or part of the muscular system beneath the skin on the face that surrounds expression muscles. A number of facelift techniques exist and are favored by different surgeons for different reasons. Most techniques have evolved over time with that particular surgeon as that surgeon gets the best results for his or her patients with his or her technique. Let's cover the options, starting with the traditional deep-plane facelift.

Deep-Plane Facelift

This is the procedure you likely imagine when you think of a facelift. The procedure boasts long lasting results, around 10-15 years. The incision and elevation is deeper, and the lift of the tissue occurs in one larger section. Ideal candidates for a deep-plane facelift have severely sagging skin and significant laxity in the face. Incisions are made above the hairline and down behind the ear. The surgeon separates the skin and the SMAS from the deeper tissues and enters the deep plane beneath the SMAS layer to loosen up tissue in preparation for lifting. The SMAS and skin are pulled upward, secured into their new position and excess skin is removed. This type of lift has mostly been replaced by SMAS facelift, as it is safer.

SMAS Lift

The SMAS lift addresses the deep layers of the face and neck as well as the superficial layers of the skin. The SMAS lift is considered a game-changer in cosmetic surgery because it allows for lift to occur higher than cheekbones and even closer to the eyes. "You need a frame to put a roof on," as Dr. Timothy Janiga describes the SMAS to his patients. The SMAS lift allows for the outer cheeks to be lifted, and consistently gives a natural result. The procedure also helps to eliminate jowls and lift and tighten the overall neck area. During the operation, the surgeon makes small incisions along the hairline and separates the SMAS from subcutaneous fat layers and soft tissue. The surgeon then elevates the facial and neck tissue upward, removes excess skin and fat, and secures it with sutures. The SMAS is the current gold standard for facelifts and gives great long-lasting natural results without as much risk as the deep-plane facelift did. Ideal candidates for this procedure have laxity in the face and neck, sagging and noticeable jowls.

OTHER FACELIFT TYPES

Mid Facelift - A mid facelift can be done with an incision at the lower eyelids or with an incision in the temple. This procedure is used for laxity in the middle of the face, but is used less now compared to other types.

Endoscopic Facelift

With an endoscopic facelift, your surgeon uses a probe and an endoscopic camera for the surgical approach. The endoscope is inserted with three incisions, enabling the surgeon to view the patient's internal facial structures on a screen. This facelift is typically used for cheek sagging and mild laxity. I would not advise the endoscopic facelift for my patients with sagging neck, as this procedure is best for specific areas of the face.

Mini Facelift

A mini facelift features a shorter incision than conventional facelifts and is a mini version of a facelift. The technique can vary depending on your selected doctor. Some techniques only lift the skin (These are sometimes advertised as "lunchtime lifts" or "30-minute mini facelifts"). The surgeon may take a section of skin from in front of the ear and tighten the skin. Results are dependent on what type of mini facelift you have. The smaller and less invasive the procedure the less result you have. If the mini that you have does not address underlying structures it usually does not last as long as a full facelift would. Some surgeons, including my husband, do a more extensive "mini" where they tighten underlying structure of SMAS. This lasts longer, typically. The ideal candidate for a mini lift has mild to moderate skin laxity and is not ready or does not want a full facelift.

Threading Facelifts

There are two different versions of a threading facelift, and we will refer to them as the "old way" and the "new way." The original thread lift procedures (the old way) were performed in the 1990s until around 2000 and involved inserting permanent sutures underneath your skin. I never got on board with this as a good option for my patients. The sutures used in this "old way" of threading lifts stayed in the patient's face forever and are close to impossible to remove. The sutures made future surgery in the areas where they are place more difficult because the surgeon has to work around the "barb wiring" and surrounding scarred tissue.

The "new way" has allowed threading to create more natural-looking result with bidirectional abilities of the sutures. The new versions also have a dissolvable suture, minimizing the risk of infection and removing the complications associated with having something in your face forever. So how does it work if the suture is temporary? After you reposition the skin with the suture, you will experience some inflammation from the procedure, and that inflammation will stimulate collagen and cause and somewhat lock you into the new position. If, for whatever reason, you cannot have a facelift and you want a lift for your 50th high school reunion in 2 months, this "new" threading method may be an appropriate option for you.

Threading is typically used for brow, neck, jawline and cheeks. This new version of the procedure is available in more than 70 countries and has been done tens of thousands of times in the U.S. At my office, we still like more permanent solutions, but there is a place for this in specific situations, and the new version is way safer than the old. This procedure boasts less downtime, less money and less invasiveness, but there is also less result. Threading can give you immediate results and can save you money, but the procedure does not replace a facelift. Consider threading a preliminary procedure before you are ready for a facelift.

Treating Loose Skin on the Neck
For years we have been doing a pretty good job of treating and protecting the face, but sometimes forgetting our neck and chest. This can lead to a difference in the appearance of the physical age of the neck and chest compared to the face. Both the neck and upper chest have recently become more of a focus with "tech neck" gaining popularity as a term, which refers to the lines that develop on your neck from increased repetitive motions from looking down at a screen. Today, there's a more comprehensive focus. You don't want a clear line between your chin and your neck (in other words, *young* looking face, *old* looking neck and chest). Therefore, maintaining your neck and upper chest compliments the effort you have put into maintaining your face.

The loose skin on the neck and the chest can be treated with noninvasive technology, minimally-invasive technology and surgery. At our office we offer all three options for patients to allow flexibility in patient preference, but also to be able to treat the mildest laxity to the most severe. From the noninvasive realm there are many options including Ultherapy®, which uses ultrasound technology, Venus, Thermage and other methods. At our office we use FORMA Plus™, a noninvasive skin-tightening device that uses radiofrequency to deliver heat to the skin and stimulate collagen and tightening. The main minimally invasive option is FaceTite™ which gives up to 30 percent tightening of the skin with one treatment. These options do offer great results, but in the case of significant loose skin around the neck, a surgical neck lift may be needed to achieve the results you're seeking.

By definition, a neck lift is usually performed with a facelift, which is one of the confusing things about a neck lift. But, you can do a neck lift without doing a facelift. Imagine that you are moving the facial tissue higher. The neck naturally comes with it, but if you do the neck alone the face is not really affected as much. A neck lift may be combined with other procedures such as facelift, eyelids, liposuction for a prominent fat pad below the chin or platysmaplasty which will be discussed below.

Treating Platysmal Banding

Another relatively common condition of the neck area is platysmal banding, which is the appearance of vertical bands on your neck (the ones that become very apparent when you clench your teeth). For significant platysmal banding, surgical intervention may be needed to make significant improvements. Platysmaplasty is the name of the surgery that addresses the platysma muscle in the neck. The surgery involves lifting or repositioning the muscles of the neck so they are not able to pull down on the skin as significantly. This is usually combined with a neck lift to remove any excess skin and possibly a facelift to address the lower half of the face at the same time. If you are not ready for surgery, or your platysmal banding is mild, neuromodulator injections (BOTOX® or Dysport®) are another option. Neuromodulators cause the neck muscles to relax so they do not pull down on the skin as much. This has a tightening effect on the neck that lasts about 3 months. You may have read about this as the Nefertiti neck lift and is a common non-surgical option for lifting the neck.

Are You Ready For A Facelift or Neck lift?

I had a patient in her 40s who requested a facelift multiple times during her BOTOX® appointments. Of course, I could have referred her to Dr. Timothy Janiga upon her first request, but instead, I explained how you can only have a certain amount of facelifts in your lifetime. If you get one at 40 you are taking away from what you might look like at 70. I encouraged her to hold off a bit, continue with her facial BOTOX®, try filler for a lift, try BOTOX® in her neck for the banding and FORMA Plus™ for some face and neck tightening. We agreed to do some tightening procedures using laser resurfacing. She was happy with these procedures and was able to hold off on a facelift for about 7 years. At 47 she did go see my husband for a consult and eventually at 49 she did have a mini facelift. She was happy she waited.

As another example, a physician came to see Dr. Timothy Janiga for a facelift and she was in her early 30s. She had a little bit of sagging, but not enough to justify a full facelift. He called me in to see her that day and I agreed with him, her face was way too youthful for a facelift. So Dr. Timothy Janiga and I worked together to create a better plan for her. She had some prominence in the jowl area or what we call *pre-jowl sulcus*. So we placed filler in each of the pre-jowl sulcus areas, which squared her jawline and improved the contours. She was extremely happy with the results and we were pleased to save her from having surgery so early. We are now 10 years later with this patient, and she does filler there about every 18 months and is still happy. No facelift yet.

What About the Mouth and Lips?

The ideal candidate for lip enhancements is a patient with a normal shape to the lip that has begun to thin over time. There are some trends out there now where very young women are enhancing the lips to the max, but this does not look good on mature women. (I could argue that it doesn't look good on anyone, but I may have to agree to disagree with these starlets). Mature women will very often come in and say, "I don't want big lips. I want *my* lips, just a little fuller." This is the type of lip filler I perform in my patients. It can be done tastefully. The aging of the lip has its own pace. I have seen young women with early lines and thin lips that have never smoked. As I have seen older women with great lip volume and no lines. This is an area where genetics plays a role. We have to remember a few things about the lip aging, not only are we losing volume in the lip itself, but the bone structure of the face that keeps the lips pouty does thin as we age. Just like osteoporosis of the arm, you lose bone volume around the mouth too. You also lose gum volume and tooth volume over time, contributing to the pinched appearance of the mouth as we age. This is an example of "long in the tooth," or the loss of gum volume that makes the teeth look longer and thinner. This is part of the same process. I usually address the lip area with multiple avenues: topicals, resurfacing and volume enhancement to get the best most natural looking results. There are several different ways to augment the lips, including lip injections and a few other procedures.

- **Filler-** There are a variety of fillers used across the world to enhance the lips. Most are soft and hyaluronic acid based in the United States. There are newer varieties that are lasting longer than before, even up to a year.

- **Fat Grafting** - With fat grafting to the lip, the lip is injected with fat harvested from another part of the patient's body. This is long lasting in most people, sometimes more than 5 years and requires a small amount of liposuction.

- **Lip Lift** - A lip lift is a surgical procedure that creates a more youthful, shapely appearance to the lips by increasing the prominence of the upper lip, lifting the corners of the mouth and decreasing the length between the upper lip and the base of the nose. Think of it as taking the lip that you have that has turned under and pulling it back out. Patients with uneven lips are also candidates for lip lifting for symmetry. Swelling and tightness is common immediately after this surgery and full results can be expected around four weeks post-surgery. This is a permanent option for patients, but you do age from there, of course.

- **Lip Implants** - Lip implants offer a more permanent solution compared to the injectable alternative. There are both natural and synthetic versions available. The implants are inserted through tiny incisions at the corners of your mouth. I do not usually recommend these, as there are so many options available to patients now. Just like eyebrows, lip styles change and these implants are permanent.

What About Nose and Chin?

Like the eyes and lips, the appearance of our chin can influence how we perceive ourselves, and therefore, how we think others perceive us as well. A recessed or "weak" chin can make a face look less symmetrical and disproportionate. A chin augmentation rebalances the facial features, improves the appearance of the jawline and can further define the neck as well. Filler and fat can be used to augment the chin as other areas of the face. If you want a permanent option there are two surgical procedures available for chin augmentation: with implants or without implants.

Augmentation with an implant involves placement of an implant through an incision underneath the chin or inside the mouth to increase the projection of the chin. Some patients may have the option of chin augmentation without an implant. In this procedure, the surgeon uses the patient's own tissue to reshape the chin and add volume. Full results for both procedures typically can be expected after 8-12 weeks.

Rhinoplasty (Nose Reshaping)

Rhinoplasty (or more commonly known as *nose reshaping or nose job*) is a surgical procedure that blurs the lines between art and surgery. The surgeon works closely with the patient to design a nose that will make the face more symmetrical and proportionate. A patient may be seeking rhinoplasty to reduce, augment or reshape the nose for cosmetic purposes. During the surgery, incisions are made inside the nose and under the nose so the surgeon can reshape the cartilage and soft tissue. Rhinoplasty can be performed along with a septoplasty, an inner nasal surgery that provides relief from the health issues associated with a deviated septum. Aside from difficulty breathing, improperly draining sinuses and chronic sinus infections, a deviated septum can also cause the nose to look crooked.

What About The Eyes?

Remember when we referred to the eyes as *the window to your age* early on in this book? The eyes speak our truths, including our age. This is why many patients looking to reduce signs of aging in their faces start with the areas around their eyes. The following sections describe different surgical options for the areas around the eyes.

Eyelid Lifts

The eyelids are the first areas that make us look tired, so it's no surprise eyelid surgery is one of the top five surgical procedures in the United States. An eyelid lift or blepharoplasty is a procedure where excess skin and tissue on both or either the upper and lower eyelids can be sculpted and repositioned or removed. The cost for eyelid surgery varies pretty widely, depending on the same things we have discussed earlier as well as whether you are doing uppers, lowers or both. While lasers or radiofrequency can be used to tighten the skin around the eyes as minimally invasive options, if there is an excessive amount of skin surgical intervention is likely needed to achieve your desired results. Note: in lieu of lower eyelid lift, some patients are candidates for filler to plump up the hollowing under the eyes and improve those dreaded dark circles.

Eyebrow Lifts

Eyebrow lifts or brow lifts, also known as forehead lifts, are a popular procedure for restoring a youthful appearance to the upper face. This procedure can be performed alone for people with a heavy brow or in addition to blepharoplasty to give them full rejuvenation. Brow lifts also help smooth out horizontal lines in the forehead and between the eyes. The ideal candidate for a brow lift has a sagging brow line that might make them look sad, tired or grumpy. The candidate may also have excess skin hanging over eyelids. While brow lifts certainly help lift the eyelids as well, some people think they need a brow lift when in fact they really need an eyelid lift, or vice versa. Your plastic surgeon will talk to you about which procedure is most suitable for your desired results. A brow lift can be combined with other surgeries of the face including blepharoplasty, facelift, chin augmentation and many others.

Surgical Procedures: Type 2 – Breast Procedures

Your face and neck might dominate your first impression, but there's plenty going on below that might be revealing your age more than you would like it to. I joke with Dr. Timothy Janiga that this might be the last year my arms can pull off tank tops (While of course that is a personal decision, I see 80-year-old women flaunting it all in tank tops). Like your face, your body is personal, and the decisions you make to work toward a more youthful appearance on different areas of your body are personal. You want to feel happy in your own skin.

Patients come into Dr. Timothy Janiga's office pinching unwanted inches in one area and asking for more *umph* or more *mojo* in other areas. No matter your lifestyle, the longer you have this body, the more signs of aging you likely have to show for it. That's aging, baby. It's a wild ride but there's no reason you have to live with all of it, especially if your appearance is compromising your happiness. Life's too short not to be body-comfortable.

One of the advantages of plastic surgery is that it affords patients the flexibility to customize their procedures to achieve their desired results. Before we dive into cutting-edge technologies and tips, I must confront the most fundamental method for achieving the body you want: proper diet and daily exercise. Wait, don't shut the book just yet! I'm writing to give you all angles of the truth for your best body, and I wouldn't be doing a very good job if I left out the basics. Exercise releases certain chemicals and hormones that boost your confidence, build muscle, burn fat and even "reverse" many signs of aging.

Between my husband and I, we can do what we do best to help you make noticeable improvements in your body shape. Taking loving care of your body is what you do best (That's why you picked up this book, right?). Healthy living is a major part of that effort. Frankly, the procedures available today do not substitute what the body wants to do naturally. Ultimately *you* change your body with smart decisions and habits for your health.

With that said, there are some areas that give you trouble no matter how well you stick to your diet and exercise plan, and that's where plastic surgery options may come in. As technologies in cosmetic and plastic surgery continue to advance, improving those trouble spots is only getting safer, more accessible and more reliable (when the procedures are performed by qualified surgeons and practitioners). More and more people are signing up for these potentially life-changing procedures. With nearly 2 million procedures performed annually, the number of noninvasive and surgical cosmetic procedures has nearly doubled since 2000, with breast procedures leading the way in popularity. Breast procedures involving surgery mainly fall in two categories: augmentation and reduction. For some, a breast augmentation would help them feel more feminine, or help them get that *oomph* back after nursing or after gravity worked its evil magic. For others, a breast reduction could help make a women feel more proportional or relieve chronic back pain and other discomforts. First up, we'll take a look into breast augmentation.

BREAST AUGMENTATION

Breast augmentation is the most popular among all cosmetic surgeries. This procedure is typically only thought of as a way for women to increase or improve the size or shapes of their breasts (or to augment one breast to better match the other). However, breast augmentation is also popular to restore breast size and shape after pregnancy, breastfeeding and significant weight loss or from basic aging and gravity. Breast augmentation mainly involves lifting, implants or both.

Breasts are an extremely personal feature of the body, so if you are considering a procedure, it is vital to be sure you and your doctor have the same expectations of your outcome. Find a plastic surgeon you feel makes an effort to understand all your needs You'll have a much better experience and you'll likely be more satisfied with the results. According to a study released by the FDA in 2011, about 20 percent of patients who received implants needed a revision or removal surgery. To avoid this, your surgeon should carefully review size expectations with you as well as implant options. Ideally, they will perform 3D imaging with you to confirm your wishes regarding size and shape. Years ago there was only one shape and you needed to choose a size, now there are multiple sizes, shapes, projections and texture options. In our office all potential breast augmentation patients are imaged with our 3D imaging software. The software takes a picture of your body and then different size and shape and projection implants can be "tried on" by the patient in her own body photo. This allows a better coordination between patient and doctor.

Am I A Good Candidate For Surgery?

Prior to your consultation, ask yourself, "Is there any reason why I shouldn't get this surgery?" Some patients who come asking for a breast augmentation simply do not qualify for elective surgery because of a history of blood clots, heart disease or stroke. Be sure that you and your surgeon are both aware of any health-related issues you may be facing prior to your procedure. Unaddressed concerns may interfere with producing the best possible outcome for you.

When it comes to breast implants, there are two main categories: saline and silicone.

- **Saline Implants** - Saline implants are filled with sterile salt water and are filled in the operating room to your desired size. Some women prefer saline implants as they feel that water is more "natural."
- **Silicone Implants** - Designed to provide a uniform shape and feel, silicone implants are filled with a soft, silicone gel and are available in a variety of shapes and sizes. Unlike saline implants, silicone implants are all pre-filled. Some implant brands carry more than 400 natural-looking, silicone-gel breast implants. Each has its own shape and feel, allowing the patient to select a customized fit with the preferred projection and feel she desires.

Breast implants are designed to enhance the size and shape of your breasts for many reasons including gaining more self-confidence, feeling more comfortable in their body or clothing, or feeling more feminine. Rarely, post-surgery, a woman may find they aren't satisfied with their breast augmentation and want to return to their original breast size and shape. To restore the previous size and shape of the breasts, a breast implant removal surgery would be done. Women are interested in these removals for a number of reasons including life partner changes, weight gain or loss, or just a general desire to have them removed.

Breast Reduction
While some women desire a larger breast size, others are literally weighed down by their "girls," causing chronic back pain, poor posture, difficulty finding clothing to fit and even low-self esteem. In this case a woman might seek a breast-reduction surgery. There are different types of breast reduction based on the amount of tissue to be removed. Discuss which type is best for you with your plastic surgeon.

Surgical Procedures: Type 3 - Body Procedures
Along with the aforementioned face, neck and breast surgeries, the cosmetic surgeries in this section can prove to boost a person's confidence, helping them feel more comfortable and confident in their own skin. For some, the surgeries mentioned here may be the only ones they ever

consider because their only points of discomfort are in these areas of the body (Think tummy tuck after having twins). The procedures covered in this section include the stomach, arms, buttocks and any area where the patient wishes to remove unwanted pockets of fat and/or cellulite (which are *not* the same thing).

ABDOMEN

Tummy Tucks

The tummy tuck surgically removes excess skin and fat for a smoother looking abdomen. Whether you've experienced significant weight loss, stubborn belly fat and skin after childbirth or you just want to tighten up your midsection, a tummy tuck may be the optimal solution for you. There are two main types of tummy tucks. One procedure moves the belly button while the other does not. The first of these, the full tummy tuck, is more involved and is for people hoping to remove larger amounts of tissue, fat and skin. At the start of the procedure, the surgeon makes an incision around the belly button, then makes another low above the pubic bone to remove any extra skin and fat. The surgeon then repositions your bellybutton and places sutures around it. You can expect 3-6 weeks of physical limitations during recovery.

The second type of tummy tuck, known as the mini tummy tuck, is less involved, using an incision along the same line as a C-section, avoiding the belly button completely. This type of tummy tuck is ideal for both men and women who may be bothered by excess skin or a small protrusion below their belly buttons. Because we make fewer incisions during this procedure, the mini tummy tuck is less extensive and has less scarring, but is only appropriate for certain patients. Similar to the full tummy tuck, recovery ranges from 3 weeks for regular activities to 6 weeks for more vigorous activities.

Whether you are a candidate for the full or mini tummy tuck, both can be performed simultaneously with other cosmetic procedures such as breast augmentation, breast reduction, liposuction, repair of the abdominal wall muscles or even a facelift or rhinoplasty.

ARMS

Arm Lift (Brachioplasty)

Sagging arms, or unkindly called bat wings, are caused by the sagging of the skin and soft tissues as we age or lose weight. It's common for people to become self-conscious about having excess skin and fat hanging from their upper arms, particularly during the skin-baring summer months. While it's not impossible to lose arm fat with proper diet and the right exercise, it can still be very difficult, especially as we get older. Tightening up the skin is even more difficult without some type of intervention.

The ideal candidate for an arm lift will have pinchable tissue and some laxity of the skin. Like the tummy tuck procedures, there is a full arm lift and mini arm lift available. For the full arm lift, an incision is made along the body side of the upper arm, which the surgeon uses to remove excess skin and fatty tissues. The incision placement is designed to be hidden under the arm. The arm lift is often performed with some liposuction, depending on how much fat needs to be removed. This allows the surgeon to better sculpt your arms to a desired shape. For the mini arm lift the incisions are mostly confined to the armpit/axilla, which is an attractive option. However, like the mini tummy tuck only some patients are candidates for the mini arm lift. You plastic surgeon will help you choose the procedure that is best for you.

You can usually return to work within 5-7 days for both options, depending on your occupation. Expect the post-surgical swelling and bruising to last for about 2-3 weeks.

Butt and Thighs

In recent years, butt lifting and augmentation procedures have grown in popularity thanks to some celebrities. We can attribute this to popular culture shifts in body images. Buttocks procedures can help to lift and create a fuller, rounder and more youthful shape. Buttocks reshaping and augmentation procedures are done with either a butt lift or with butt implants. The thighs can also be reshaped with a thigh lift. Butt and thigh procedures are often coupled with liposuction or other body contouring procedures.

Options For Non-Surgical Contouring

If you are looking for a non-surgical option for arm contouring, there are two main options. First, a contouring procedure can be done with BodyTite™, which is a non-surgical, minimally invasive procedure that can help contour the arms in a single office visit. The area can be treated in approximately 1-2 hours. Second, there are procedures such as BodyFX™ and FORMA Plus™ that are noninvasive options requiring multiple treatments.

Butt Lift and Lower Body Lift

Traditional butt lift technique is done for massive weight loss patients or other patients that have significant redundancy of the skin of the buttocks. In this procedure the buttocks are physically lifted higher by making an incision on the lower back and upper portion of the buttocks to remove excess tissue and lift the area.

The traditional lower body lift usually involves tummy tuck and buttocks lift. This procedure involves making an incision along the circumference of the beltline (around the front and back of the body). Commonly, this procedure is done for people that have had massive weight loss through surgery or healthy life changes and have maintained their current weight for over 6 months. As with most surgical procedures, recovery takes at least 3-6 weeks but can be longer with a full body lift in some cases.

Buttock Implants

Like breast augmentation with silicone implants, buttocks implants use silicone implants to increase the size of the butt for a lifted, rounder and more youthful shape. Buttocks implants are a alternative for patients who would like a larger derriere, but lack excess fat deposits that would be used for fat transfer procedures. To perform the procedure, an incision is made below the cheek near the top of the thigh. The surgeon then creates a pocket either below or above the muscle and inserts the implant. Recovery takes about 3-6 weeks.

Brazilian Butt Lift

A trend that's really skyrocketed over the past couple of years is the Brazilian Butt Lift. The look—which increased in popularity around the same time celebrities such as Kim Kardashian and Sofia Vergara came onto the scene—is achieved by surgically taking fat from areas such as the abdomen, flanks or thighs through liposuction and transferring it into the buttocks. This procedure has seen a 200 percent increase over the last couple of years. The Brazilian Butt Lift is generally done at the higher area of the buttocks to give it that desired lifted appearance. This procedure takes about two hours, and recovery can take between 2-4 weeks. Using fat grafting rather than an implant helps give a more natural look and of course the fat is your own healthy tissue. Because the surgeon uses your own fat from a different party of the body, the fat will feel and act like it's in its natural place. However, like all fat in our body, it changes with the aging process. You can consider a Brazilian Butt Lift a semi-permanent surgical procedure whereas butt implants are permanent unless you have them removed.

SURGICAL FAT REDUCTION

Liposuction

Liposuction, sometimes called *liposculpture* or *lipo*, is the well-known procedure for sculpting and removing unwanted fat from parts of the body including, stomach, buttocks, abdomen, thighs and neck. Liposuction is the second most common cosmetic procedure in the U.S. after breast augmentation (and up 5 percent since 2016). [3]

When I tell my patients that liposuction isn't technically meant to assist in weight loss, that it is a sculpting procedure, they're usually surprised. Liposuction is meant to be a tool to aid your body sculpting goals if you are already close to a healthy weight. Trying to achieve massive weight loss via liposuction is a risky proposition. This is because liposuction, like some other fat reduction procedures, has a limit to the volume of fat that can be removed. You might recall the story about Kanye West's mother dying after liposuction. While we don't know the full story, we do know that she died after the day she had a significant amount of liposuction. When you remove a tremendous amount of fat, you are also removing a lot of electrolytes, which your heart needs. Having too many or too large of a procedure in a day is dangerous for this reason, among others. When you're losing a ton of fluids, your body doesn't have time to compensate and replace those electrolytes.

The ideal candidates for liposuction are at or near their ideal weight and have stubborn areas of fat deposits. For example, patients with pear-shaped bodies typically have small amounts of excess fat deposited in the hip area even though they have a flat stomach and thin arms. Patients with an apple shaped body may have thinner legs but hold excess fat deposits in the abdominal or flank areas. Even though people with these body types seem to try everything, they still can't seem to lose the weight. For these situations, liposuction is optimal. Before the procedure is performed, it is a good idea to discuss with your doctor your current weight, any recent weight loss or gain, dietary habits, and exercise habits so you have a holistic approach toward creating the body you desire.

The gold standard of modern liposuction uses the technique known as tumescent liposuction to dilute the fat before it is removed. Tumescent liposuction infuses salt water along with epinephrine and local anesthetic solution into the fatty tissue before it is broken down and sucked out. A thin tube called a cannula connected to a vacuum is then placed in the tissue and the surgeon moves that cannula back and forth sucking out the fat deposits.

Liposuction itself is pretty standard, but there are ways to augment the liposuction for different body types that require a little more finesse. Gynecomastia (unwanted male breast tissue) is a great example of this as this is denser tissue. There are three ways to deliver heat to the fat to assist with liposuction when needed: laser-assisted, ultrasound, and radiofrequency.

- **Ultrasonic Assisted Liposuction (UAL)** uses ultrasonic waves to melt the fat as it is sucked out.

- **Laser Assisted Liposuction** is a form of liposuction that uses lasers to melt the fat before it is sucked out.

- **Radiofrequency Assisted Liposuction (RFAL)** uses thermal energy (radiofrequency) to assist with liposuction. The radiofrequency liquefies the fat, making it easier for the cannula to suck it out. This is the type we use in our office because we feel it gives the most tightening.

These additions to liposuction give moderate to significant tightening, depending on which on you choose. Not all body areas will need or require these additions, but it is nice to ask about them if you want to know if you are a candidate for this additional part of the procedure.

Most liposuction procedures need to be done in an outpatient surgical facility, but small areas like arms, submental fat pad and inner and outer thighs can be performed in the office under local anesthesia. There is usually some bruising and tenderness of the area for one to three weeks afterwards. Liposuction patients can often return to deskwork within two days. Patients can expect bruising and swelling with this procedure.

The cost of liposuction depends on which areas of the body are treated, with larger areas like the abdomen costing more than the small submental fat pad.

Considerations For Your Operation
For the best results, you need a board-certified plastic surgeon operating on you at an accredited surgical facility. You should control all the variables you can. Your surgeon should be technically skilled, have plenty of experience with this procedure, have great attention to detail and keep your best interests at top of mind at all times. You can and should ask to see previous work and even talk to a previous patient of the plastic surgeon if that would make you feel comfortable. At our office we have a list of patients that have had specific procedures that are willing to talk to future patients about their experience.
It's important to remember surgery doesn't end when you wake up. Post-surgery is an ongoing process of healing and recovery. There will generally be some discomfort after surgery, and there will often be questions you forgot to ask or ones you already asked but need clarification on. Each patient's recovery process is different, so you want a surgeon who has

a wide range of experience with patients who have different pain level, length of recovery and overall post-op journey. The best surgeons will make themselves available to answers these questions before and after your procedure.

Risk-Benefit-Cost

Risk Level:	Benefit Level:	Cost:
High	High	$$$$

Risks and Precautions

Dr. Timothy Janiga puts a lot of emphasis on making sure his patients understand the potential risks of surgical procedures before the big day. Cosmetic surgical procedures have many of the same risks as medical procedures, with the general exception that, for cosmetic procedures, it is common practice for the patient to be healthy. Conversely, in medical procedures, that is not always the case. To reduce the risks of surgery, please read Chapter 13: *Choosing The Right Dermatologist or Plastic Surgeon* carefully.

Other Concerns & Treatments in Youth And Beauty

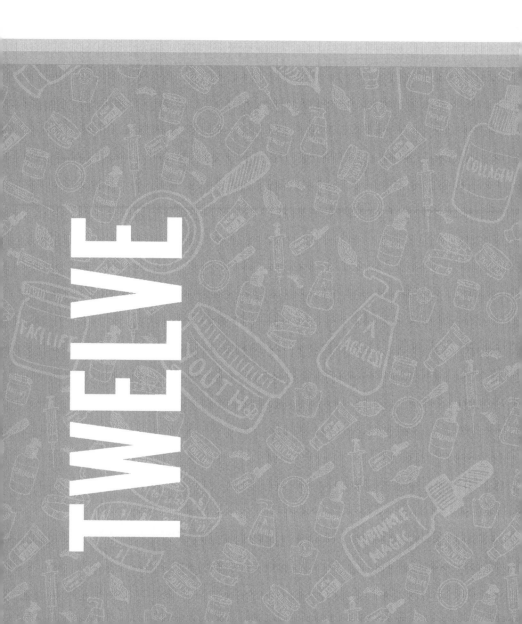

TWELVE

OTHER CONCERNS & TREATMENTS IN YOUTH AND BEAUTY

Cellulite Treatment

Cellulite is usually described as cottage cheese-like ripples beneath the skin (or orange rind bumps, for my cottage cheese lovers). Both thin and heavy people can have cellulite, as cellulite is the collision of skin and fat, of which we all have both. This bumpy look is caused by fibers, known as septae bands, which pull on the skin and tether the tissue down. The fat sticks out between these fibers, causing the fat to bulge. Cellulite is caused by a number of genetic, hormonal and physiological factors, though it's not an indication of poor health. This is why people of all shapes and sizes can have cellulite.

Data shows that 80-90 percent of post-pubescent women have cellulite, and yet we look at it as a condition, something unwanted. I personally think this partially has to do with the smoothing out done in Photoshop®, among other tricks of mass marketing so we think that there are more people in this world without it than with it, this is just not true. Despite the entirely common nature of cellulite, it remains unacceptable to most women.

At-Home Cellulite Masking Tip

Have you ever noticed people with darker skin types seem to have little to no cellulite? This is because darker skin hides cellulite better. If you're light skinned, I'm not advising extra hours in the sun. But if it really bothers you, find an at home tanning cream or spray tan. The change in the optics does seem to help.

Cellulite treatment requires different procedures than fat reduction does. Wanting cellulite gone is almost always an aesthetic choice, and there are minimally invasive as well as noninvasive ways to treat cellulite. The noninvasive treatments that are available should be used for patients with mild to moderate cellulite. The most effective, in my opinion, is a device called BodyFX™ that has no downtime, very little discomfort and good results. This is a radiofrequency-based device that uses suction, heat and bursts of radiofrequency to break up the fibrous bands that contribute to cellulite. As with all noninvasive technologies, multiple treatments are required as well as maintenance treatments. The two minimally invasive treatment devices should be considered for those with severe cellulite. Tumescent anesthesia is used to numb the area and then a probe is inserted underneath the skin to break up the fibers that attach. There a variable yet appreciable results with both of the machines that are currently available, called Cellulaze™ and Cellfina®, and you will see results within a few weeks and these last a few years.

Topical creams and topical devices that shine on the skin have not been shown to decrease cellulite in clinical trials. If your cellulite really bothers you, consider one of the devices available: BodyFX™, Cellulaze™ or Cellfina®. That being said, topical treatments will not hurt you so if you think that cream helps you, go for it!

Massage

Massage is commonly advertised as a way to treat cellulite; however, there is no evidence that massage gives any lasting improvement for cellulite. This is the same for creams, oils and detox methods; but if you feel that it's working for you, go for it.

Bleaching Creams and Pigmentation Treatment
The most common way to topically treat pigmentation is with a bleaching cream. Most bleaching or "fading cream" you buy over the counter are exfoliants, which means the active ingredient is either salicylic or glycolic

acid most of the time. It might help your pigmentation look a little better in the short term, but it won't make significant long-term changes. The physician dispensed bleaching creams are pigment inhibitors. Most of them work two ways to prevent production of pigment, and to decrease pigment that is already formed. Our pigment-producing skin cells (melanocytes) secrete a pigment ball into the skin, or melanosome, and the bleaching cream inhibits production of these melanosomes while also decreasing pigment under surface of the skin. Besides bleaching and brightening products, retinoids help also by decreasing pigment production (You'll want to get the proper concentrations for your skin from your dermatologist). In my practice, the patients I see want to use a multifaceted approach to remove pigment as fast as possible, with sunscreen, laser (such as IPL spot lasers) and lightening products.

The two main categories of bleaching or brightening products are hydroquinone and hydroquinone free. Why the separation you ask? Well, there has been some controversy surrounding the ingredient hydroquinone after some reports showed that hydroquinone can cause permanent darkening of the skin and has been shown to cause cancer in rats. After consideration by the FDA they determined that the reports of problems with hydroquinone were so rare that they were not going to ban the ingredient. I advise my patients (and think about it for my children and myself) in this way. If you have a medical condition that needs bleaching this is a good temporary medication for improvement of that pigmentation. It should be used with sunscreen and in as limited amounts as possible under physician supervision. Then hydroquinone-free medications should be transitioned in with sunscreen and lasers for long-term maintenance.

While the hydroquinone free products are physician-dispensed, hydroquinone and retinoid are on the pharmaceutical grade side of the spectrum and you will need a prescription. You can buy 1 percent hydroquinone over the counter, whereas the prescription concentration is 4 percent or higher. I can also compound 12-30 percent if needed for shorter periods of time. The higher concentrations, closer to 30 percent, are the super versions of hydroquinone that Michael Jackson used to bleach the rest of his skin when he had vitiligo. I have not given 30 percent concentration to anyone that was not trying to combat the medical condition of vitiligo, but it is possible though very specialized. The higher the concentration the higher the possibility of side effects, as with most things. For cosmetic purposes, we usually stay between 4 percent and 12 percent.

Hair and Sweat Reduction

Hair and sweat are two body features we always seem to be messing with. Fortunately there are more methods of managing hair and sweat than ever before. While it is still not possible to completely remove hair in one magical session or completely eliminate sweating, there are methods to reduce both.

First let's talk "removal" versus "reduction." Removal implies that all hair or sweat will be gone, reduction more accurately shows that hair and sweat will be reduced. All treatments (except for electrolysis, which is used for hair removal) currently available for sweating and hair are *reduction* treatments. None are *removing*. Reducing hair or sweating is ideal for those with excessive sweat or unwanted hair.

Laser Hair Reduction

Laser hair reduction (LHR) uses laser light technology to target the pigment in the hair shaft and deliver heat to the area, which destroys the follicle. LHR is considered a reduction treatment because it can only treat hair in the growth cycle. As only some of your hair is in the growth cycle at one time, LHR requires a session of treatments to achieve desired results. Each part of the body has hair with different growth cycles and a different percentage of hairs in that growth cycle. For this reason, LHR for upper lip hair is done every 6 weeks while legs are about every 3 months to target hair at its various growth cycles. Once patients understand this, they look at LHR differently and are more likely to complete their treatment sessions in my experience.

Data shows that most of the hair can be removed with about five treatments with the new devices, but it is possible for some hair follicles to regrow or for you to develop new hair in the area and require ongoing treatments, this is especially true for the facial hair as women age. Be cautious of anyone who tells you they can permanently remove all of the hair in any body area forever, as this is frankly not possible. Most reputable laser hair reduction providers will let you know that most areas will require maintenance over time, possibly a treatment or two every couple of years to keep the area smooth.

DECREASE SWEATING

miraDry® is a popular procedure for permanently decreasing underarm sweat by 86 percent. This low risk procedure has proved well worth it for many people. Though, one of the most common questions we get is whether the body will sweat more in other areas if you reduce the sweat under the arms. There's no need to sweat (not that you'd want to!) there is no evidence that this would happen. The underarm is home to less than one percent of sweat glands on your body, so getting rid of some of them will not harm your overall body's physiological balance or ability to cool itself. miraDry® is a heat-based device.
The underarm area is numbed and suction-based heat is delivered to multiple zones under the arm. After the numbing most patients feel a slight warming sensation but no real discomfort. If miraDry® doesn't sound like your thing, you do have other options, like BOTOX® medication and prescription antiperspirants. But, miraDry® is the only option that permanently decreases sweat.

If you have tried prescription pills, prescription-grade antiperspirants as well as neuromodulator injections and would like something more permanent, miraDry® may be right for you. Look for a board-certified dermatologist or plastic surgeon's office to have this done, as there is a small chance for infection and you want to be somewhere that can take care of you before, during and after the procedure.

If you have sweaty palms, neuromodulator injections into the palms and fingers can be a life-changing procedure. I have a patient who is a nurse, she has such excessive sweating of her hands that the sweat actually pools in her exam gloves and flings around when she takes them off. With neuromodulator injections into the hands every 6-9 months, she is more of a normal sweating level. This allows her to work, not be embarrassed, and remain sanitary. She is an extreme case, but if you are prone to excess sweating of the hands, see a board-certified dermatologist or plastic surgeon for these injections as these are more complicated and come with different risks and techniques than BOTOX® for crow's feet.

If you would like to exhaust all your options before you do injections, there are prescription medications, prescription antiperspirants and Iontophoresis. Iontophoresis is a technology that has been around for quite a while, and it works for many people. This procedure uses a water bath with positive and negative charges to reduce sweating in the hands and feet. The sweat glands use little ion channels to secrete sweat. You submerge your hands into it for a few minutes, a few times a week, and it reduces sweating of hands and feet by disrupting the ion channels. This and the other medications require a prescription from a physician. I find this option great for teenagers with sweaty hands, and I even have a few teenagers currently using it. Teenagers typically don't want the shots and parents aren't particularly fond of having their kids on unnecessary medications. This is also a good option for those that prefer a more natural approach, avoiding chemicals and prescription medications, or for those who want the convenience of treatment at home.

Methods for removing hair temporarily - There are many methods for removing hair temporarily, and most people have to find the method that works best for them by trial and error. Some methods may irritate your specific skin, while others can cause you to form hair bumps. Try a few different methods (though not at the same time) and remember that different parts of your body may respond differently. Skin sensitivity on the arms and legs is different than the underarms and near the bikini line, for example. Tolerance to certain temporary hair removal methods can also change as you get older.

Shaving/Dermaplaning – Most people know what shaving is of course, but dermaplaning is a variety of this that is worth discussing. It is done by a qualified esthetician usually in a medical spa type setting with a hand held blade. The blade is run over the entire surface of the skin removing "dead skin" and any hair. This technique is great for those people with that peach fuzz type hair as it does a great job removing it. It also takes away the top layer of skin that needs exfoliating and allows makeup to lay nicer and medications to penetrate better. Dermaplaning lasts anywhere from a week to 3 weeks depending on the rate of growth of the peach fuzz.

Chemical Depilation – This procedure includes the over-the-counter creams you apply to cause the hair to fall out at the root. These used to be just for body hair, but at least two companies have facial versions now. If you have sensitive skin test these in a small area that is less visible before using all over. These last longer than dermaplaning or shaving, as it takes the hair at the root lasting up to 3 weeks in some people.

Waxing / Sugaring – Waxing and sugaring are two popular hair removal procedures performed by estheticians in many spas and salons. The goal with waxing is to use soft, hard or even chocolate wax to remove the hair from the follicle and damage the follicle with the intention of stopping it from producing hair in the future. Follicles are resilient though, so it can take several sessions before you notice areas where hair growth is decreased. The results of a single wax, which takes most hairs out at the root, can be up to 3 weeks.
Sugaring is a process by which a paste made of sugar, citric acid and either water or honey is applied to the skin to remove hair. This is often the route for people with more sensitive skin that cannot wax, as it is all-natural and the paste is usually applied at a lower temperature than wax.

Does Shaving Cause Hair to Grow Back Thicker?

You might have heard rumors that shaving causes your hair to grow back thicker, but there is no real data to say shaving changes the coarseness of your hair at all. Hair is naturally changing as you age and waxing and shaving doesn't make it coarser.

Hair, Sweat And Hormones

For those going through hormonal changes, you might be experiencing an increase of sweating or unwanted facial hair in areas it's never been before. Your primary care physician or gynecologist should evaluate these conditions for their cause before treating the end results of sweating or unwanted hair. Once you have determined that there isn't anything medically to do, then you should treat the symptoms. For example, menopause is a normal change of life in women that bring along hormone changes, sweat changes and hair changes. What's really happening is the type of hair present on your face is changing. Before menopause, women's facial hair is mostly vellus hair, or what we call "peach fuzz." When women enter menopause we begin to grow terminal hairs, or those coarse, dark, beard-like hairs. This is not an "abnormal" occurrence, but it is undesired by most women—hence laser hair reduction.

SCARS, STRETCH MARKS, AND KELOIDS

Understanding Scars

A scar is a medical term for the disruption and reformation of collagen in an area of trauma. Any trauma that reaches the dermis and disrupts the collagen can form a scar including acne, burns and cuts. Anytime you cut the skin, there is a scar. Much (if not most) of scar formation has to do with the specific circumstances of the person and genetics (Think about those certain people who get keloids from a simple ear piercing, whereas the rest of us have no problems). Some work can be done to improve the aesthetic of a scar. For example, certain stitches can be used to improve the appearance of tummy tucks scars to reduce tension.

It is extremely important to follow your scar care instructions after your procedure. These will be given to you by your surgeon and are not to be disregarded. If you want your scar to heal properly, that is. You can think of post-surgery scar care as maintenance step. The better you take care of your scar, the less money you will have to spend later on doing revisions if you are not happy with it.

Of all the products and procedures on the market, my opinion is that resurfacing with lasers or radiofrequency does the best job of remodeling a scar for better appearance. There is also evidence that treating fresh surgical scars with silicone sheeting improves the way scars look after surgery. This sheeting is not to be confused with silicone cream, stretch mark creams or over the counter scar creams. Silicone sheeting comes in strips that you cut to fit the size of the incision and lay over the length of the scar. It is usually safe for people allergic to latex or adhesives, but make sure to check labels if you have a history of this problem. The theory behind why silicone sheeting has been shown to improve appearance of scars is thought to be due to the application and distribution of pressure across the incision. In our office we include these silicone sheets with all of our surgery packages to ensure that it is available to our patients right after sutures are removed.

There is some evidence that neuromodulators injected around a fresh scar on the face can improve the appearance of that scar. A study was conducted years ago where they took the length of scar from a Mohs surgery and injected the neuromodulator BOTOX®. [1] They found the scar healed in a cleaner, line. The theory behind using a neuromodulator is that the muscle inhibiting properties changes the muscle contraction around the scar, keeping the muscle from pulling on the stitches. Because this is not covered by insurance it is not commonly done for scars after skin cancer excisions on the face. It is also not really possible to do for an abdominal scar for a tummy tuck because of size and expense. But, it does underline the point that your surgeon will make to you after a procedure. Rest and do not exert yourself too much afterward so your incisions can heal with the best results possible.

When looking at scars and treating them, notice that both of the above strategies are on fresh, newly formed incisions. These work best for new and healing scars. If you're 60 and you don't like your tummy tuck scar from 20 years ago, that's more difficult to work with because it is a fully formed and mature scar. I'd say it's even a labor of love. Improvements are possible, but you have to decide if what science can give you at this time is worth it to you. You should discuss this with your doctor to help you find out what is best for your specific situation.

Acne Scarring
Acne affects 85-90 percent of teenagers and up to 15 percent of adults. While not all acne leaves scarring, the large cystic lesions with the deep component are the most likely to leave scars. The smaller whiteheads and blackheads are less likely to leave significant scarring. The best way to avoid acne scars is to prevent them altogether, which is why it is important to receive care for your acne when it starts. While some people are more prone to scarring than others, there's no real way to predict who is and who is not going to scar, so it's best to make a commitment to acne and scar prevention. First, make an appointment with a board-certified dermatologist to help you manage your acne. Second, keep your hands off your face and resist the urge to pick and squeeze. Lastly, be patient and realize that a lot of people have acne and not all acne leaves scars, but the scarring is on the radar of every dermatologist. When I meet with my patients, I tell them that my one job is to try to make sure that they do not get one more scar on my watch.

There are a few different types of acne scars that can leave unsightly depressions in the skin, and as we age and our collagen breaks down they can become even more noticeable. Treating acne scars looks different depending on the type of acne scar. To improve this deep type of scarring you must be able to affect collagen down deep. With lasers and some types of fillers the appearance of acne scars can be dramatically reduced.

Icepick and Rolling scars usually form after large, deeper cystic acne lesions. The deep inflammation disrupts the collagen and causes the dents and irregularities in the skin. Ice pick scars are small and almost look like little holes in the skin. Rolling scars look exactly like they sound. When magnified the skin looks like rolling hills with depressions and elevations in the areas that have been affected.

Boxcar scars are square or box-like. They are formed from repeated picking at a healing acne lesion. The scab is removed multiple times and the underlying area is squeezed and manipulated. I honestly do not think that these types of scars form on their own. In my opinion they form only from manipulation of lesions over and over.

Techniques to treat the different scars vary by distribution and type. The TCA CROSS method, subcision, filler, dermabrasion, deep collagen stimulation lasers and radiofrequency can be helpful for scarring. If you have a combination of these scars, as most people do, then fractionated resurfacing treatments might be best for you to start with. As you can see, acne scarring is not as straightforward as one would think. It is best to be seen by an experienced dermatologist to make the best plan for your type of scarring.

It's important to remember treating acne scars is like treating any scar. It takes time, patience and an understanding that the goal is to get the best scar you can get.

Hyperpigmentation From Acne

Hyperpigmentation is also a common result of acne-induced inflammation and is technically not a scar as it is not permanent. Hyperpigmentation will fade naturally if you avoid the sun and can be treated with bleaching and brightening products if you would like them to fade a little faster than the body allows. It is essential to protect hyperpigmentation with sunscreen, as sun exposure can worsen the spots.

Keloids

Keloids are overgrown scars that mushroom out from the original smaller scar as they heal. Keloid scars are most common on the chest, back, shoulders and on the lobes after ear piercing. There's no way to predict a keloid if you've never had surgery before. Keloids can be genetic and are more common in certain nationalities like Asian and African. If you have a history of keloids make sure to inform your surgeon.

Stretch Marks

Stretch marks are medically called striae and occur after unusually fast growth, weight gain or during pregnancy. Stress marks are extremely common, in fact most people get them over the course of their life. The most common areas for stretch marks are the abdomen, breasts, butt and thighs. They usually start as red or purple and can be raised and itchy as they start. Over time they become lighter in color (almost white and shiny) and look slightly wrinkled. With excessive stretching of the skin, the collagen, elastin, and fibrillin are damaged, like a scar. Who gets stretch marks and who doesn't is only controllable to a certain extent. Your genetics will play a large role. I have a lovely young female patient that had her first child around 21, started at a very healthy weight, and only gained 19 pounds with her pregnancy. She got stretch marks from her breasts down to her knees. This was worst case I have ever seen with such a small weight gain. Her stretch marks are clearly 100 percent out of her control and have more to do with her genetic makeup.

The best way to prevent stretch marks in pregnancy is to follow your doctor's advice and try to keep the weight gain to just a few pounds a month. The current guidelines recommend weight gain closer to 25 pounds for pregnancy in a normal female (I gained 62 pounds with my second pregnancy so I may not be a great example here). If you have teenagers, encouraging them to maintain a healthy weight can help try to prevent stretch marks in adolescence. However, not much can be done to prevent stretch marks in those that are genetically predisposed or grow 9 inches in one year.

Unfortunately, despite all the preventative treatments on the market for stretch marks, like creams and lotions, there isn't any evidence that they can prevent stretch marks. That being said, they will not do any harm, so if your friend gave you the "cream that prevented stretch marks for her," go for it. As long as you are not allergic to one of the ingredients, it may not help, but it won't hurt.

Treatment of Stretch Marks
As we discussed there are two different phases of stretch marks: the red/purple development stage and the white scar-like mature stage. At the beginning stages of stretch marks when they are red or purple you can use vascular lasers that target red to decrease the intensity of the redness if that

bothers you. This will have some improvements on the color immediately, and on the collagen long term. When they are in the white scar-like stage, you can use collagen stimulating products and resurfacing to improve the appearance, like scar treatments reviewed earlier.

The two topical products that have shown improvement of the scar like white stretch marks are topical tretinoin (retinoids) and hyaluronic acid. Tretinoin helps to stimulate collagen and elastin while hyaluronic acid brings hydration to the skin making the stretch marks look better. Chemical peels have also shown some improvement in the appearance, but this might only be temporary.

Collagen-stimulating radiofrequency treatments and lasers are the gold standard for treatment of stretch marks and some are even approved by the FDA for this. Multiple treatments are required, but you can improve the appearance of the white scar like stretch marks by up to 50 percent. Other options that have some benefit (albeit less than resurfacing) include microneedling with or without PRP, microcurrent and galvanopuncture, as anything that stimulates collagen can help.

Butters and Oils for Stretch Marks

Every pregnant woman lathers herself up with a cocoa butter or vitamin E oil to prevent stretch marks. Unfortunately, the few studies that have looked at the moisturizers (cocoa butter, shea butter, vitamin E, olive oil or almond oil) and stretch mark prevention did not show any improvement in the number of stretch marks formed during pregnancy. But again, if you like it and feel that it may help you, go for it.

The bottom line is that anything that penetrates to the deeper layers of the skin and affects the collagen in the dermal tissue does seem to make some improvements once formed, but the gold standard for treatment of stretch marks is still resurfacing.

I See My Mother's Hands!

When you look at small child's fists you will notice they have little, adorable mounds of fat on the top of their hands. Then you look at an older hand and you can basically see the entire finger bone run all the way to the wrist. Many women have come into my office alarmed that their hands are beginning to look exactly like their mother's hands. While there is certainly some genetics at play here, there are also environmental factors. We have usually been less mindful about skin care and sunscreen on our hands than we have been for our face. Because skin on our face and hands are typically the most sun-exposed skin on our body, factors that age the hands are similar to what age the face. You get photoaging, collagen and elastin reduction, brown spots and even volume loss. If you are fortunate enough not to have laxity on your face yet, but you feel that the skin on your hands is showing your age, there's a way to test it. Pinch and pull up on the skin of your hands, and you might notice it stays up. It's called tenting, and it's a sign of laxity on the hands.

The hands need the same protection and maintenance as the face, including sunscreen, anti-aging treatments and emollients. Personally, I use emollients on my hands at night and I wear sunscreen on my hands whenever sun exposed. I regularly receive laser treatment for brown spots on the tops of my arms and hands, and when I am done putting retinoid on my face, I rub a little into the top of my hands.

Treating Aging Hands

Like all areas of the skin, it is best to follow the prevent, maintain and improve method when treating the hands. Starting with prevention and protection, make sure you're wearing sunscreen on your hands during prolonged sun exposure. That includes driving. As far as maintenance goes, you can use the same active ingredients in your topical treatments meant for the face on your hands too. Our skin on the top of the hands is like paper. It's almost as thin as eyelid skin. Just as I advise my patients to use both face and body treatments on the more delicate skin on the neck and chest, you can follow the same method for effective anti-aging hand treatment. Personally, I use extra emollients on my hands at night. When I am done putting my anti-aging products on my face, I rub the rest into the top of my hands. I also treat the brown spots on the top of my hands once per year. If you're like me and have a dominant sign of hand aging that is bothering you, then it may be time to seek treatments. When we treat a hand for aging, we suggest eliminating brown spots first with brown spot lasers like IPL or other pigment laser. Next would be to replace volume in the hand with fat or Radiesse®, which is an FDA-approved filler to rejuvenate the hand. It is made of calcium hydroxyapatite and does a great job revolumizing the hands. Fat grafting is another option replenishing some of those fat mounds for a younger looking hand. Fat grafting to the hand is similar to the process of fat grafting to other areas in that you must undergo liposuction from a donor area and then have it placed in the top of the hands.

Leave No Toe Unturned - Scanning for Skin Cancer

Skin cancer screening is an important part of every dermatologist job. Bob Marley died from untreated melanoma on his toe. When I do skin checks on people, I will look in between toes, behind your ears, in your scalp and on your nails. If you have polish on the nails all the time, make sure to take it off for your skin check, and once in a while between skin checks just to see any abnormalities.

Choosing the Right Dermatologist or Plastic Surgeon

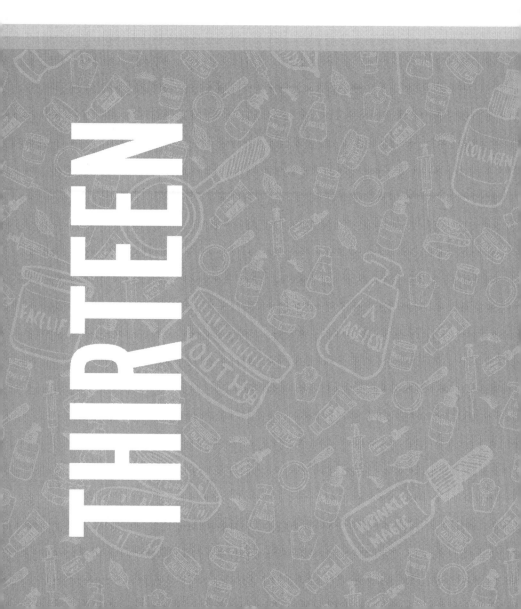

THIRTEEN

CHOOSING THE RIGHT DERMATOLOGIST OR PLASTIC SURGEON

Your relationship with your dermatologist or plastic surgeon should be a long-term one. As the patient, you are the ultimate decision maker, so you should always feel comfortable enough to speak up when you have questions or concerns. It's an open conversation.

When you have a doctor who listens to your wishes (and really hears you), you gain an advocate. When I'm with a patient speaking about a potential procedure, I make sure to ask what my patient understands about this procedure so I can help fill in the gaps. Together you and your doctor will make major cosmetic and medical decisions. Go into their office having a clear understanding of your role in the process. This doesn't mean you need to become an expert in cosmetic medicine. That's not your role, as the right doctor will guide you through all your surgical and noninvasive options, carefully explaining recovery information and the pros and cons of all options. You should be an expert at gaining and assimilating that information.

COSMETIC PROFESSIONALS AND QUALIFICATIONS

Note: Rules and laws of governing bodies are different in each state, and these explanations are meant to be general. Please check with your medical, nursing, or cosmetology board in your state for specific guidelines for these categories of providers.

Esthetician or Esthetic Technologist (1 year of training) - Estheticians perform various skin, hair, and nail-care treatments, makeup applications, facials and full-body skin treatments.
Certifications Necessary:
- Esthetician certification from a cosmetology school is 9-12 months
- State licensure by the cosmetology board in your state

Laser Technician – Most states do not require schooling or certification and do not have boards. Laser Technicians are trained by the laser company or by the physician in the office on that device. Because of this there is no regulation of training hours. If you are having laser with a laser technician that is not certified as a nurse, a nurse practitioner, or a physician assistant, it is fair for you to ask what certification they have and how much training on that laser device they have.

Cosmetic Surgery First Assist (1-6 years of training depending on type) - A cosmetic surgery assistant works closely with surgeons during pre-op and in the operating room preparing tools and providing other surgery assistance. They also help with administrative duties and discharge paperwork. Most cosmetic surgery assistants have experience in other healthcare fields and are certified by either the nursing board as a nurse surgical assist, the PA board as a physician assistant, or as a certified first assist. These certifications are monitored and governed by the state, the operating facility, and your surgeon. A surgery assistant cannot currently operate in any state without a physician.

Aesthetic Nurse (4 years of training) - Aesthetic nurses, or cosmetics nurses, work with dermatologists and plastic surgeons and are educated in laser theory, pharmacology, injectables, infection control and camouflage cosmetics.
Certifications Necessary:
- RN degree
- RN nursing certification exam
- State licensure by nursing board in your state

Aesthetic Nurse Practitioner or Physician's Assistant (6 years of training) – Nurse Practitioner or physician assistant (PA) that works with a dermatologist or plastic surgeon. This practitioner has a higher level of education than an RN and may prescribe medications, see patients without a physician and manage patients.
- Bachelor's degree, 4 years
- Masters degree in either nursing or PA school, 2 years (though it is likely in 2022 this will be required to be a 4-year doctorate program)
- NP or PA certification exam
- Certification by the state board of nursing as a nurse practitioner or by physician assistant state board

Nurse Anesthetist (6 years of training) – Nurse anesthetists are nurses that receive special training after nursing school to administer anesthesia for surgery. Guidelines in each state differ as to the required amount of supervision by a board-certified anesthesiologist, so check with your state for guidelines.
- Bachelor's degree in nursing, 4 years
- One year of clinical experience in acute care
- Nurse Anesthetist Master's degree, 2 years (though it is likely in 2022 this will be required to be a 4-year doctorate program)
- State board certification

Anesthesiologists (13 years of training) - Anesthesiologists are professionals in anesthesia theory. Board certified physician anesthesiologists have years of training in anesthesiology and emergency situations that arise during surgery.
Certifications Necessary:
- Bachelor's degree, 4 years
- Medical school: M.D. or D.O., 4 years
- Residency in anesthesiology, 4-5 years
- Certified by The American Board of Anesthesiology (ABA)

Dermatologist (12 years of training) - A dermatologist is a doctor who specializes in the health of skin, hair and nails. After receiving a Doctor of Medicine degree, dermatologists must complete a residency program in dermatology, which includes education in general dermatology, pediatric dermatology, dermatologic surgery, cosmetic dermatology, complex medical dermatology and dermatopathology.

Certifications Necessary:

- Bachelor's degree, 4 years
- Medical degree: M.D. or D.O., 4 years
- Internship in medicine or pediatrics, 1year
- Residency in dermatology, 3 years
- Certified by the American Board of Dermatology (ABD)

Surgeons - Cosmetic surgeons (and surgeons with a plastics or cosmetic fellowship) work to reconstruct and reshape the human body to either enhance a person's looks or restore their appearance prior to a traumatic injury, disease or failed operation. All surgeons receive a Doctor of Medicine degree and undergo a residency and fellowship. Below I've broken out the different surgeon designations and explained their necessary certifications.

***Plastic Surgeons* (14-18 years of training)** – Plastic surgeons repair, reconstruct, or replace physical features of the human form. Aesthetic surgical principles are used for both cosmetic changes and for reconstructive changes. Plastic surgeons are certified to operate on the head, face, neck, breasts and body, and plastic surgeons can pursue a subspecialty in any of these areas.

- Bachelor's degree, 4 years
- Medical degree: M.D. or D.O., 4 years
- Plastic Surgery Residency 6-10 years depending on program
- Certified by the American Board of Plastic Surgery

***Oculoplastic Surgeons* (12-13 years of training)** - Oculoplastic surgeons receive certification through the American Board of Ophthalmology and are required to complete a fellowship after "eye residency" in order to perform cosmetic eye surgeries.

- Bachelor's degree, 4 years
- Medical degree: M.D. or D.O., 4 years
- 4 years residency, 1 year cosmetics fellowship for cosmetic eye surgery
  Note: Because the ophthalmologist cosmetics fellowship is specific to eye surgery, these surgeons are known as oculoplastic surgeons and perform cosmetic surgery only around the eyes.

ENTs or Facial Plastic Surgeons (13-14 years of training) - Ear nose and throat doctors or ENTs are certified by the American Board of Otolaryngology and are required to complete a "facial plastics fellowship" after residency to be considered facial plastic surgeons.

- Bachelor's degree, 4 years
- Medical degree: M.D. or D.O., 4 years
- 5 years ENT residency then 1 of fellowship in cosmetics for nose and face
  Note: Because the ENT cosmetics fellowship is specific to the nose and face, ENTs with a cosmetic fellowship are usually called facial cosmetic surgeons and cosmetic procedures are traditionally confined to the nose and face.

Professional Experience

Experience goes a long way! The average physician has 10,000 to 20,000 hours of direct patient care contact prior to treating their very first patient on their own. In contrast, in descending order nurse practitioners or physician assistants with a master's degree have approximately 850 to 1,500 hours, RNs about 600 hours, medical assistants about 200 hours and estheticians somewhere around 100. Once each certified professional finishes their training, they then gain additional experience by treating patients or clients. Cosmetologists that specialize in hair move into a salon as an apprentice for a year and then work their way up. The woman who cuts my hair was an apprentice for a year and then she moved up based on the number of years of experience she has. Once she reached seven years at her salon she became "master," the highest designation.

The point with explaining the different training and certifications necessary to hold certain titles is to help you choose your professionals wisely, to know their credentials, and know what that credential means. If you choose to have medical or cosmetic services performed, make sure that the person has thousands of hours of experience after their training in that specific field. For example, the nurse practitioner who works with my husband and I has her master's degree and is a certified nurse practitioner; but in addition she has more than 15 years of experience with her physician supervisor in lasers and injectables. If you do the math, 40 hours a week times 50 weeks a year is 2000 hours. It will take at least 5-10 years for a certified nurse practitioner or physician's assistant to reach the 10,000-20,000 hours of clinical experience treating patients as a physician has when they finish their residency. Choose wisely, choose experience and choose education. Knowing how much experience your provider has accumulated in certain areas of specialization will help you choose the most appropriate provider for ideal results and safety.

Your Face Is My Face
Let's turn the table for a second. As a cosmetic professional, there's a level of humility at which you have to admit what you don't know, and there's so much you come in contact with in this field to realize what you don't know. Throughout my residency and on through my career (even to this day), I see conditions in which I don't know what the patient's *best* option is right away. I may call a colleague that I trust and run the case by them, look up a condition in the literature, or just think about it for a couple of days. These situations remind me that, as a professional in this field, you have to have enough knowledge to know what you don't know. Any reputable doctor will admit this. After you've been seeing patients professionally for 10 to 15 years, you gain more and more knowledge, but there's always something that will require more learning. It comes down to knowing I will do everything I can to provide the right care my patients require—even if that means referring them to a different specialist and losing them as a patient. Knowing what you don't know is just as important as being awesome at what you do.

As a patient, you put your trust in the hands of your doctor, and that trust goes both ways. Cosmetic changes are deeply personal, so reputable cosmetic practitioners take great lengths to ensure patients feel the doctors are providing the same care they would expect for themselves. When you select a board-certified dermatologist or plastic surgeon with a specialty in cosmetics, you're choosing to work with someone with years of experience in cosmetics and plastic surgery. This doctor will have the expertise needed to guide you in the direction that most fits your desires, your need for discretion and your availability for recovery time.

Having surgery isn't a decision to be taken lightly. Having that date pinned into the calendar triggers a rush of questions you deserve to have answered by someone with enough depth of knowledge and experience to inspire complete confidence. This is a partnership to achieve the look you want for your face and your body. Way before you ever commit to any operation, please take the time to find a surgeon who listens attentively to your questions and answers them with confidence and clarity. Hopefully after reading this book you have a few more questions to ask of them.

Together, with your trust and your doctor's expertise, you will come to an agreed set of expectations for the results of your procedure. It's important for you to fully understand what can and cannot be done during your procedure. Being armed with this sort of information can help you plan accordingly prior to surgery.

Addressing Complications
Both technology and technique in cosmetic medicine are continually advancing, minimizing risk and making incredible results more accessible than ever. But *minimal risk* does not mean *no risk*. We will never be able to eliminate all risk when dealing with procedures or surgery. This is something we all know but like to tuck away into the corner of our minds. With the guidance of your doctor, expectations will be set based on your medical history, your goals and your standard of "normal." If you have any medical problems, allergies, or even a recent major lifestyle change (like quitting smoking), your surgeon will know whether you can have the surgery now, need to wait or are not a candidate at all. No matter how badly you want your selected procedure, never lie or hide information from your doctor.

Knowing the risk of complications is real, so ask your provider how they would address complications. Sure, this question may feel a bit out of your comfort zone (They are the expert, right?). If your provider chooses not to answer this question, find someone who will. It's better to know now rather than later. Of course there are the rare cases of procedures that cause unforeseen complications, the .001 percent possibility. You have the right to know exactly how your doctor will handle that rare moment. Asking about your doctor's complication game plan is just one of 10 crucial questions you should practice asking your doctor. What are the others? We're glad you asked.

Be Your Best Advocate Checklist

1. **Am I safe?** This is always number 1. Are you in a clean environment with sanitary conditions (biohazard containers, gloves, hand sanitizer)? Is each member of the staff polite and qualified to perform all the procedures they are performing? If something rare or unexpected happens—say you have an allergic reaction to an injection—you want to be confident they can save your life. Most reputable places have name tags for employees with their title on them, so each patient can read without having to ask what level of training the person in front of them has. It should be open for discussion, not a secret.

2. **Are you board-certified by the American Board of Plastic Surgery?** This is a national standard and should be the first question you ask your plastic surgeon. While residency contains cosmetic training and a test to be board certified, there are practicing doctors who did not take their boards. Be warned: addressing board certification with your surgeon can sometimes be a complicated conversation. Start by asking if they are specifically board-certified by the American Board of Plastic Surgery, and your surgeon should be able to give a clear, definitive answer. In some cases, you may come across a physician who is board certified in a specialty not directly related to cosmetic surgery, but advertised as such. Some may even possess a title in "cosmetic surgery." Though, be aware that most of these are not nationally recognized by the Board of Plastic and Reconstructive Surgery. Board-certified physicians are accredited by the American Board of Plastic

Surgery and are required to complete a rigorous residency program specifically designed for plastic surgeons. Be your own advocate.

3. **What are the complications of this procedure?** There are complications to all procedures, so if your doctor claims there is nothing to worry about with your procedure, be wary. If I personally cannot manage 99 percent of potential complications for a given procedure, I will gladly refer the patient to someone who can. All my reputable colleagues would do the same. You should also have a clear understanding of who will take care of you if there are any complications. Is there a doctor that will evaluate you if you are sick in some way after this or will you have to go to the ER, urgent care or your primary doctor (who are likely less qualified to manage cosmetic complications and products as they do not do these every day).

4. **What is your medical title?** This is a completely appropriate question that any medical professional should feel comfortable answering. Before any procedure you should know whether they are a medical doctor, a nurse practitioner, a physician's assistant, an RN, a qualified esthetician or just someone with a syringe offering champagne with your service (Don't laugh, this really happens). In our office, everyone wears a nametag that clearly displays their specific designation(s).

5. **What did you complete your residency in?** You wouldn't want a pediatrician doing your heart surgery, so why would you want a doctor with training in another specialty doing your facelift operation? Be confident your doctor did their residency in the field they say they're practicing. Some doctors like otolaryngology (ENT), and ophthalmology doctors can do training and become board certified for certain cosmetic surgeries after finishing a "facial plastics" fellowship. This can be a little confusing, so just don't assume white coat means doctor.

6. **Are you a member of the American Society for Aesthetic Plastic Surgery?** This specific certification is only given to board-certified plastic surgeons after they have accumulated significant cosmetic experience. Each physician's cosmetic experience is reviewed by an independent group of established cosmetic plastic surgeons, and if the criteria have been met, they will become a certified member

of the American Society for Aesthetic Plastic Surgery. Having a clear understanding of your doctor's past professional experience will help you feel confident, not only in their ability, but also in the results to be achieved. Request before and after photos of their work for the specific surgery you are doing.

7. **If I have photos taken of me, did my doctor's office ask for permission to use those photos?** When you ask to see photos of a doctor's work, they received permission from the patient to share these images. Knowing what counts as a HIPAA violation is a great way to be your best advocate for any cosmetic or medical treatment, procedure or transaction. Only medical professionals have to abide by HIPAA, that means estheticians and hair stylists at a salon do not. We have a HIPAA officer at our office and a HIPAA compliance plan we keep in a fat binder at the office. You should also ask how this facility protects your medical information. They should be held to the highest standards if they are performing procedures on you.

8. **Do you provide discounts through discount finder sites like Groupon, FatWallet, or Living Social?** I do not have a reputable colleague that uses these sites. Period.

9. **Does your surgeon operate in an accredited facility?** For your own safety, facilities need proper accreditation for authorized procedures. If the worst happens, it is also helpful if your doctor has access to a hospital nearby. My husband, as a board-certified plastic surgeon, will only do procedures in an accredited outpatient surgery center to ensure the best care for our patients.

10. **I'd like to get a second opinion.** Any reputable provider won't worry about you getting another opinion and will recommend another provider for you to see for that opinion if you would like. If the provider is hesitant to refer you, that is a warning sign (but it can also mean their ego is abnormally large). Ask if you can speak to another one of their patients that has had this procedure with them. Most of us have patients that are willing to speak to other patients about procedures. If your surgeon says you don't need surgery, it is likely you do not, but a second opinion is fine.

FINAL THOUGHTS

Throughout this book we have confronted the cultural and personal influences that contribute to our understanding of beauty and aging standard, and occasionally drive us up the wall. We have walked down the skin care aisle, examined the ingredients lists of common products, and distinguished essentials from trends and fluff.

We have reviewed physical aging from bone to skin, and you now have a comprehensive overview of skin issue classifications and phototypes. We've identified the various dominant features that concern us most in cosmetics and aging. Together we've climbed The Ladder, looking more closely at the treatments and procedures available to address these dominant features at each step. We've peered behind popular brand names for a clearer picture of the processes that give you results. From topical at-home treatments to surgical fat reduction procedures, we have confirmed there is risk and reward every step of the way, and I hope these truths have become more transparent (and less intimidating) to you.

- **In the skin care aisle** – Now with your knowledge of the six topical essentials, you are equipped to navigate beauty and anti-aging aisles with a sharp eye and a cool head. You can identify active ingredients, spot a money pit from a mile away, dodge the distractions and select products that specifically target your dominant concerns.

- **At home** – You can step away from the 10X mirror and trust that you are doing what is best for your personal needs. Protect your skin and prevent further damage with sunscreen and antioxidants. Maintain your skin with moisturizers and regular exfoliation methods. Repair and improve your complexion with retinoid treatment and growth factors.

- **In the dermatologist's or plastic surgeon's office** – You are the ultimate decision maker, and your dermatologist (or plastic surgeon) is your partner in making informed decisions that align with your individual needs. Your doctor may certainly be the expert in their field, but you are ultimately the expert on *you*, and that information is key to getting the best results from any procedure. Use this *Be Your Own Best Advocate Checklist* to answer pressing questions and concerns. And remember, you are not alone in thinking these things! Your uncertainties are common, though the proper solutions are unique to your individual needs.

There are many tools, stories and scientific facts throughout this book that were designed to assist your pursuit for personal cosmetic improvement. If you get anything from this book, I hope you feel more confident making informed cosmetic decisions on your own behalf, acting as your own most trusted advocate, and tackling the skin care aisle without losing your lid. After all, you are the authority on your cosmetic goals. Next we will confront some deep-seated myths about the effectiveness of procedures and certain expectations with these procedures.

16 MYTHS: SKIN AND HEALTHCARE PRODUCTS, TREATMENTS, COSTS AND RISKS

1. Plastic surgery is only for celebrities and people who want to look "perfect."

Many people who explore cosmetic surgery begin their consultation saying, "I don't want to look like one of those plastic, frozen dolls." In all honesty, there are very, very few people who do. Our understanding of cosmetic surgery has been skewed by the extreme cases we see on television and in Hollywood. As it is with many cultural standards, the coasts are what we like to call outliers, and there are more people who live in these urban areas who prefer more dramatic procedures: huge lips, large breasts, cheeks lifted to the heavens, etc. That's not the "norm." Those cases are also more obvious out and about than someone who just got some BOTOX® to manage some forehead wrinkles.

The majority of people who are looking into a surgery do so with the intention to live happier lives, and that typically means a little trimming here, a lifting there, and as natural looking as possible. In fact there are probably several people at work, in your cycling class and at the grocery store that have invested in a procedure, and you wouldn't even know it. Wanting to look your best is not vain or shallow. In fact most people do want to look their best.

While it is an overgeneralization to associate cosmetic procedures with celebrities and the wealthy, it is common for those in the public eye to consider surgery before, say, someone who spends most of their time working in a lab or in front of a screen. This has more to do with the cultural expectation placed upon them. Let's be honest, there are not that many haggard looking female movie stars able to get jobs in their chosen profession.

The same notion applies to all women compared to men, who are disproportionately represented in cosmetic surgery. But it's not that men didn't think of getting their wrinkles minimized or their waistline shaped before. The stereotype has made them uncomfortable, hesitant to go sit in a room with only women. According to the American Society of Plastic Surgeons, 2015 was the first time that men accounted for more than 40 percent of breast reduction procedures in the United States (You've come a long way, guys). [1] Men usually come in for noninvasive procedures like microdermabrasion, CoolSculpting®, soft tissue fillers and BOTOX®. Surgical procedures include nose reshaping, eyelid surgery, breast reduction in men, liposuction and face lifts. Men and women alike can have plastic surgery.

2. Cosmetic surgery can "fix" my imperfections.
Cosmetic surgery has advanced dramatically over the last 20 years. We are able to reconstruct breasts, improve the facial structure of children with cleft palate, and even perform cranial reconstruction after traumatic scenarios like the procedure performed on the young activist Malala Yousafzai after she was shot. We can help severely obese patients get closer to a healthy weight, and we can improve the curves of people post-pregnancy. What we cannot do is reverse time or make your hard-earned signs of aging vanish during your lunch hour. We cannot 'fix' things, but we can improve the appearance of the issues that bother you.

An important and less publicized part of successful procedures is the healthy expectations of the patient. Dr. Timothy Janiga and I put a lot of emphasis on helping our patients expect realistic outcomes. We find advertisements for certain procedures can project unrealistic (though believable) expectations, so we use technology and case studies to show our patients what is possible. In our experience, this process is key to patient satisfaction. We also encourage our patients to avoid words like "fix," "perfect," "gone" and "disappear" when communicating expectations. When the patient and provider are on the same page, the patient is far more likely to enjoy their results. Science says we can't make a 60-year-old look like a 30-year-old. Modern plastic surgery is meant to improve the appearance of features that bother you, not to alter you completely. Though, many of our patients feel like new people after moderate changes!

3. Blood and Gold are the new "it" ingredients, so they must be better than what already exists.

We explained these two trends in Rung 2 of The Ladder (*Facials, Peels and More*). The gist: they are trends. The "vampire" facelift is called so because it involves the patient's own blood drawn from their arm, spun, and then applied to the face in order to stimulate collagen, therefore "lifting" the skin. The other trend is the "gold facial," which includes the application of a facial mask made with 24-karat gold foil. While both the vampire facelift and the gold facial are effective and impressive treatments with a hyped-up status in the media, they are not right for every person and every budget. In fact, there are several options that incorporate similar science. You can get great results without the hyped brand name that your local superstar got this week. Ask your provider what is available to you and what works for your specific needs.

4. Can laser hair removal cause cancer?

There's been some sensationalized talk around laser hair removal and cancer. There is no evidence that this is true. Laser hair reduction has been performed for over 20 years safely and in experienced hands.

5. Do silicone implants pose serious health risks?

With any surgery, there are risks and potential side effects. Both saline and silicone-filled implants have an outer shell made of medical-grade silicone. Saline implants are filled with water and silicone are filled with medical grade silicone. They both come with a company warranty of about 10 years. Most women replace their implants with new ones after 10-15 years.

Do silicone implants cause lupus? For 14 years the silicone version was removed from the market for fear of systemic conditions like lupus. There has since been large studies done showing that there is not an increased risk of lupus with silicone implants. They have been back on the market now for years as a great and safe option for patients.

What about mammograms? If you have heard that mammograms are less sensitive in women with implants you are correct. There is some evidence that implants decrease the amount of breast tissue that is visible by 10 percent if they are under the muscle and possibly 30 percent if they are on top of the muscle. That being said, there is no evidence that women with implants who get breast cancer have a later diagnosis, larger tumors, worse prognosis or stronger likelihood of death. So, even if it decreases visibility on mammogram, this does not seem to translate to a worse outcome for women diagnosed with breast cancer. Most facilities now ask if you have implants prior to your mammogram and do some special views to help increase the amount of tissue that is visible. All women should schedule mammograms annually or more often if your doctor recommends, do your self breast exam every month, and report any changes in your breast to your doctor.

The improved techniques and advancing technology have made breast implants more accessible. The information available supports that silicone implants are safe when monitored in a medical environment. Breast implants provide serious emotional and psychological benefits to women of all body types and socioeconomic statuses. Naturally small-chested women have undergone surgery to make their body more proportionate. Others have enjoyed increased self-esteem with breast implants. If you are considering breast augmentation surgery, discuss the procedure thoroughly with your doctor.

6. Can I get fat reduction procedures instead of a tummy tuck?

A tummy tuck is the gold standard procedure for improving the waistline, but it is a surgical procedure, which may not be ideal depending on budget or available downtime. The recent advances in cosmetic medicine have made it possible to offer non-surgical methods, such as CoolSculpting® or BodyTite®, to reduce fat deposits in the midsection (and other areas of the body where localized fat accumulates). So, how do you know what is best for you? The best way is to discuss your expectations and cost to benefit ratio of each procedure with your surgeon based on your anatomy and desired goals.

- In general, CoolSculpting® is designed to decrease an individual fat pad by 25 percent with each treatment. Plus, it gives a little tightening of the overlying skin. If you have localized fat deposits and good skin tone, this should work for you.
- BodyTite® will remove fat really well and tighten skin about 30 percent, so if you have mild skin laxity and fat this may be for you.
- A tummy tuck removes excess fat and skin and tightens the underlying structures. If you have significant fat deposits and moderate to severe skin laxity a tummy tuck is likely your best option.

At the time of consultation your surgeon will perform an examination to help you decide which procedure will be most beneficial to you. At our office we provide all three categories of procedures, from noninvasive to minimally invasive to surgical. Make sure your provider can offer the full spectrum.

7. Will injectables move around my face?
Rest assured, injectables do not have travel plans of their own. While BOTOX® can diffuse and filler can migrate under certain rare circumstances, for the most part injectables stay beneath the injection site. Because BOTOX® is a liquid form it can diffuse slightly; though precautions can be taken to minimize this and help is stay in place. A number of factors are thought to influence the diffusion of BOTOX®, including the dilution or dosage of the product or the muscle selection. For these reasons it is highly advised to receive injections from a qualified clinician.

While it is uncommon, filler can migrate a bit. I have only seen this happen a few times in 15 years. Hyaluronic acid fillers are biocompatible and biodegradable, so in the few cases I have seen we have dissolved the product without an issue.

8. If you want high-quality products and care, you have to fork out the cash.
Yes and no. A lot of my patients spend thousands of dollars more than necessary, over the course of a lifetime, on products that are not right for their skin. Before you hand over your credit card, invest in a little education about your options. Learning what you need, how much you need and where to get it can help you make more informed decisions about what's worth spending money on, and what's just trending, overpriced or useless. There will be some treatments and procedures with a bigger price tag, and you and your doctor will decide together whether that is a worthwhile investment.

In this book we review products that are worth spending money on and others you can save money on. A retinoid that costs $20 won't give you the same result as the prescription strength for $70, and investing in the prescription strength will save you money down the line. But I won't let you spend money on a $90 cream that claims you'll lose 10 years off your face in 6-8 weeks. You don't need brand-name products to get the results. You need the high-quality, active ingredients (and the proper concentrations) for the best results.

9. I want a facelift, but I can't afford one. Will this cream that calls itself "facelift in a jar" be a good substitute?
Look, as much as we wish and hope for a magical cream that can give us the results of a facelift, it simply doesn't exist. A true facelift is the gold standard in cosmetic surgery. It is a procedure where the surgeon makes an incision and removes excess skin and tightens underlying structures. Creams are meant to supplement your regiment, not replace the higher rungs on The Ladder.

10. Is it OK to receive certain noninvasive procedures from a non-certified practitioner with the proper equipment?
If a license is needed before a person can perform a procedure of any kind, then you should only go to someone who is licensed.

Never perform a procedure yourself or accept treatment from an unqualified practitioner, even if they are qualified to do other procedures. Although it can be tempting to walk into a space that offers steep discounts on filler or lasers, I highly discourage you from cutting corners with cosmetic treatment of any kind. In fact I would stop you right at the door if I could.

I would bet you know someone who has had laser hair removal, and I would also bet that you or someone you know has heard of someone being burned during treatment. Laser hair removal devices have certain settings that need to be adjusted depending on skin type and hair pigment. With laser hair removal, it is more risky if you have a tan, and the settings will need to be adjusted. Patients with darker skin (Types 4-6) need a totally different type of laser to have it done at all. This is because the laser is targeting pigment in the hair, and darker skin confuses the laser, thinking the pigment in the skin is the pigment in the hair. My friend who is of Indian descent went to have laser hair reduction done and she was burned on the stomach from the procedures. Five years later she still has little brown squares where the lasers burned her. The laser isn't intuitive, so a qualified practitioner must change the settings to the needs of the patient. No matter what procedure you are signed up for, you must be confident the practitioner is qualified to use whatever machinery needed. In addition, remember there are side effects possible with every (and any) procedure. As your own advocate, ask if your practitioner is qualified to help you if one of these happen to you. If not, who will? Is there a physician on site?

11. Can household or natural skin remedies take the place of noninvasive and surgical procedures?
If you are skeptical of certain over-the-counter cosmetics and prefer to use natural and household remedies, I have no problem with that. However these masks, scrubs and moisturizers are mainly for daily care and preventative use. They cannot replace the heavy lifting done by noninvasive and surgical procedures but can be a nice addition to your maintenance regimen. An interesting exception to this is antioxidants. You can get antioxidants in creams, foods, masks and supplements. However you get them is fine with me, as they are an essential in anti-aging and overall skin care.

12. Is it safe to buy a single ingredient like a retinoid or hyaluronic acid online?
With the overflow of information online encouraging innovative at-home solutions and a DIY approach, taking control of your aging never felt so accessible. If you know the ingredients you need, then you can find them in over-the-counter products and prescription-strength cosmeceuticals with a quick search. The primary issue here is not whether you can treat yourself at home, it's whether you should. Just because you can buy something online, doesn't mean it's safe to put on your skin. Even if you are a certified esthetician or other professional in the cosmetic industry, there's no guarantee you will get what you paid for. If you plan to purchase a product online, be 150 percent positive.

- The product was produced in the United States.
- The concentration is appropriate for at-home cosmetic use for *your* skin type.
- The product is sealed upon arrival.
- You actually know how to use this product.
- The product comes from a reputable company that has transported it and stored it at an acceptable temperature as not to inactivate the ingredients or cause contamination.

If someone has to have a license to do a procedure, it's usually best if you have it done in one of those places. When it comes to deep chemical exfoliants and other treatments, let the pros handle it.

13. I'm on a BOTOX® budget and have a friend doing filler for half the price. Is this safe?
Buying a sweater for 75 percent off is a steal to be celebrated. Receiving a cosmetic procedure for less than the standard price is not. If you're getting injectables from an unlicensed practitioner or a friend who has access to some product solely to save money, you're thinking of an aesthetic procedure as cost instead of an investment. Money and safety are not interchangeable, and I advise you to err on the side of caution. As a dermatologist with medical large volume purchasing power, a single syringe alone costs me upwards of $300-500 to buy from the company. If a friend is giving filler treatments for $285, that should raise an eyebrow

(and not in a good way). There is clear danger of expired, low quality or fraudulent product that you are about to inject into your face.

I am aware of an injector in our area who injects BOTOX® and filler at house parties around town. First, she does not carry the education or certifications necessary to be a nurse. She has been arrested on multiple accounts, but she continues to inject BOTOX® and fillers at house parties. As a community we have done what we can to educate our patients and report her to authorities, but at times you just have to know that if it seems too good to be true. It likely is. Based on what you know from reading this book, you can protect yourself from situations like this. Keep yourself safe by always having medical procedures done in a medical office with a medical professional—one that will take care of you before, during and after the procedure.

14. Can I really get liposuction in 30 minutes?
Can you get a facelift in a jar? (See Question 9). The same logic applies here. I'm sure you've seen the Med Spa windows with signs boasting "Lipo on your lunch break," but I would not be doing my duty as a doctor if I told you that it was safe, let alone possible. The average liposuction procedure takes 2-3 hours. While flirting with the idea of losing 20 pounds during your lunch while your coworkers scarf down sandwiches at their desk might be irresistible, it really is too good to be true. Minimally invasive procedures like CoolSculpting® and Sculpsure® are options for quick fat reduction procedures—35 minutes per area without prep time, massage, and check in and out. However, surgical results take longer than your lunch break to achieve.

15. Should I buy collagen pills/creams?
I tell my patients to save the money and buy a steak instead. There is not enough data to suggest consuming collagen by pill helps your skin to produce it. The data we do have states it is chemically impossible for collagen pills to be ingested, broken down by the stomach, put into the bloodstream and put back together as collagen in the skin to replenish lost collagen in your face. At this time it is not worth the money, but you never know what the future holds, so stay tuned.

16. I'm doing everything and NOTHING is working. What am I missing?

Recently I had a patient who had struggled with a rash on her feet for 8 years. She had seen the ER, her primary care doctor, and her daughter who was a nurse. She had been applying and soaking in so many different things and nothing worked. The first thing we did was halt all treatment, then I handed her an occlusive moisturizer for her feet. We discussed the difficulty to diagnose or make a recommendation with all these products and chemicals on board. Being that she was a willing patient, she went home and did what I said—basically nothing. She came back 3 weeks later and was completely cured. We ended up saving that patient over $300 a month on prescription medications, not to mention doctors visits. She was free of her condition for the first time in almost a decade, by doing nothing! But sometimes doing nothing is everything.

It's common for clients to come in and show me all the products they use daily that don't work. Sometimes patients are trying 20 or more new serums, creams, cleansers and other cosmetics on their face in a week. Upon consultation I could find that maybe you're doing too much and you need to do nothing for a while.

Whether you're desperate to find a cure-all for your sensitive skin or you just love trying to new cosmetics, I recommend controlling how often you introduce a new cosmetic product to your regimen. If you are going to use something, use it for 4-6 weeks before giving up and moving on to the next thing. Even prescription products take 4-6 weeks to work.

APPENDIX

Special Populations and Considerations

There are some skin conditions that may determine the beauty products and treatments that you should and should not have. Here we will address the most important ones, in the sense that a person with any of these conditions could have direct repercussions if they are not mindful of skin treatment limitations. If you have these or any other medical conditions please make your provider aware prior to any cosmetic lasers, procedures or surgery.

Psoriasis

Psoriasis is a chronic inflammatory skin disease that confuses the immune system into thinking it should grow skin cells more rapidly. This causes red patches to form on the body that are sometimes painful or itchy. While many patients have psoriasis on less than 3% of the body, there are others that are quite severely affected. No matter how severe, the psychological effects related to this disease have a major impact of quality of life. Psoriasis patients have been shown to suffer from depression, low self-esteem, negative body image, metabolic syndromes, cardiac disease, as well as frustration and anger from lack of effective treatments. Psoriasis is an immune disease that affects the overall health and effectiveness of the skin barrier.

1-2% of the population is affected with psoriasis and those people should take special care when deciding on what type of cosmetic procedures to have and with whom. If psoriasis is active, you may have open areas of skin on your body that make you more susceptible to infection in the areas treated with cosmetic procedures. Open areas of skin should not be treated with any types of laser or injectables. Psoriasis is also known by dermatologists to exhibit a phenomenon called Koebner Phenomenon. This is where any trauma to the skin can bring out new lesions of psoriasis, this includes "trauma" from injections and laser treatments. If you have psoriasis you should take caution to make sure your provider is aware of your condition and takes the proper precautions when treating you.

Vitiligo

Vitiligo is a condition where the body attacks its own pigment cells (melanocytes), causing them to stop functioning. This leaves white patches in the affected area. For this reason, it is considered a type of autoimmune disease. The condition is found in people of all ethnicities but is usually more noticeable in patients with darker skin. Like patients with psoriasis, patients with vitiligo can exhibit the Koebner Phenomenon and should make their provider aware of their condition.

Atopic Dermatitis (Eczema)

Atopic Dermatitis or "the itch that rashes" as it is known in the dermatology community, is one of the most commonly treated skin conditions in dermatology. Eczema is a reaction of a defective skin barrier. Within the barrier, there are misfiring keratinocytes, which allows environmental irritants to do their damage on the immune system. This causes the definitive itchy rash that can sometimes burn. It is most often found on the neck, arms, lower legs, and lower back. Some may also get it on the eyelids and behind the ears. Like most inflammatory skin diseases, treatment for Eczema starts with hydrating and calming the skin. Then your doctor will rule out dietary or environmental triggers. Common treatments include corticosteroids and calcineurin inhibitors. If you have eczema you may need to avoid certain topical antiaging medications or at the very least be monitored more closely so please make sure your provider is aware if you have a history or active eczema.

Acne

What's in a breakout? Why do our faces look swollen some days or patchy on other days?

Following the prevent, maintain and repair method is a bit trickier for some people because acne is often caused by factors that are difficult or impossible to control, like hormonal changes for example. We're all familiar with the hormonal acne that troubles us in our teens, but many people experience adult acne too. This can be extremely frustrating, especially when you're also dealing with signs of aging and collagen is less abundant, making scars less likely to heal as best as they could. Post inflammatory hyperpigmentation can appear when people develop blemishes, cysts or nodules. People with darker skin get dark spots after acne, while people with lighter skin might get red spots, even if they didn't pick. If you have acne there are certain precautions taken with topical medications as well as with certain laser procedures. Please let your provider know if you have a history or are currently affected by acne. *For more on treating acne and common procedures, see Rung 2 of The Ladder* (Facials, Peels and More*).*

Lupus

Lupus is a systemic (or whole body) autoimmune disease. It can affect skin, kidneys, eyes, joints, blood, liver and most other organs. Most lupus patients have skin sensitivity to sunlight and special precautions should be taken with these patients if they are receiving light-based treatments like Intense Pulsed Light or Broad Band Light. In addition, they have a base of inflammation in the body and may have increased risks during surgery or other procedures.

Lichen Planus

Lichen Planus is an inflammatory skin condition that is less common than psoriasis but manifests with purple or red spots on the skin. They are usually scaly and also exhibit the Koebner phenomenon.

Herpes Simplex Virus

Cold sores (herpes) are a viral infection that recurs a few times a year usually around the mouth. Cold sores are contagious and can be activated by trauma to the area and can spread to damaged or open skin. If you have cold sores or herpes on the face or neck make your provider aware before you receive any procedures, injections, or surgery to that area so they can give you a prescription medication to help keep any breakouts under control.

Body Dysmorphic Disorder

Most of us have a feature we are not particularly fond of, whether it's our nose, our eyebrows, or our love handles--that's a major part of being human. While we've all got our "imperfect" something, it usually doesn't preoccupy our daily thoughts.

For people with Body Dysmorphic Disorder (BDD), their imperfection is everything, they do not see past it. In fact, an imagined or slight flaw might consume them for hours each day. BDD sufferers are incapable or otherwise refuse to believe others when they say there is no flaw, or that they look better than they think they do. Unfortunately, the imperfection can never really be perfected; it is an ongoing problem because it is rooted in his or her perception of the flaw, not the objective aesthetic feature. For this reason, and others, your surgeon or dermatologist typically has your medical records and performs a formal assessment of your expectations from a procedure. Your doctor wants to give you results that align with healthy expectations.

Depression and Anxiety

Depression and Anxiety are both common conditions in the United States. Neither are necessarily reasons not to be treated cosmetically, but both should be under good control with your primary doctor or psychiatrist prior to any cosmetic procedure, laser or surgery to achieve your best outcome.

REFERENCES

CHAPTER 1

[1] Zebrowitz LA, Fellous JM, Mignault A, Andreoletti C. "Trait Impressions as Overgeneralized Responses to Adaptively Significant Facial Qualities: Evidence from Connectionist Modeling" C Pers Soc Psychol Rev. (2003; accessed Aug. 2017) 7(3):194-215

[2] Zebrowitz LA, Montepare JA. "Social Psychological Face Perception: Why Appearance Matters". Soc Personal Psychol Compass. (May 1. 2008; accessed Aug. 2017); 2(3): 1497.

[3] Rentschler I, Jüttner M, Unzicker A, Landis T. "Innate and learned components of human visual preference" Current Biology, (June 14 1999; accessed Aug. 2017), 9:665–671

[4] Penton-Voak IS, Burt DM, Perrett DI. "Investigating an Imprinting-like phenomenon in humans." Evolution and Human Behavior. (Jan. 2003; accessed Oct. 2017) Volume 24, Issue 1, Pages 43-51 (https://www.ehbonline.org/article/S1090-5138(02)00119-8/fulltext)

[5] Rhodes G. "The Evolutionary Psychology of Facial Beauty". Annual Review Of Psychology. (Aug. 11, 2005 accessed Oct. 2017) Vol. 57:199-226 https://www.annualreviews.org/doi/10.1146/annurev.psych.57.102904.190208

[6] Thornhill R, Gangestad SW. "Human Facial Beauty" Human Nature (1993) 4: 237. doi: https://doi.org/10.1007/BF02692201

[7] Little AC, Jones BC, "Evidence against perceptual bias views for symmetry preferences in human faces." (2003; accessed Oct. 2017) Proceedings of the Royal Society of London B, 270, 1759-1763.

[8] Pallett PM, Link S, Lee K. "New 'Golden' Ratio For Facial Beauty." Vision Research. Jan. 25, 2010; accessed Nov. 2017); 50(2): 149 doi: 10.1016/j.visres.2009.11.003

[9] Di Dio C, Macaluso E, Rizzolatti G. "The Golden Beauty: Brain Response to Classical and Renaissance Sculptures." (Nov. 21, 2007; accessed Oct. 2017) http://journals.plos.org/plosone/article?id=10.1371/journal.pone.0001201

[10] Langlois JH, Roggman LA, "Attractive Faces Are Only Average." (Mar. 1990; accessed Oct. 2017) Psychological Science. Dept. of Psychology University of Texas Austin Vol 1. NO.2

[11] Thornhill R, Gangestad SW. "Human Facial Beauty" (1993; accessed Oct. 2017) Human Nature 4: 237. doi: https://doi.org/10.1007/BF02692201

[12] Folstad I, Karter AJ. "Parasites, bright males and the immunocompetence handicap." (1992; accessed Oct. 2017) American Naturalist. 139:603–622.

[13] Zebrowitz LA, Montepare JA. "Social Psychological Face Perception: Why Appearance Matters." (May 1, 2008; accessed Oct. 2017); Soc Personal Psychol Compass. 2(3): 1497. doi: 10.1111/j.1751-9004.2008.00109.x

[14] Penton-Voak IS, Perrett DI, Castles DL, Kobayashi T, Burt DM, Murray LK, Minamisawa R. "Menstrual cycle alters face preference" Nature (1999; accessed July 2017) 399:741-742

[15] Lucintel. "Growth Opportunities in the US Skincare Market." (Nov. 2013; accessed Jul 2017) http://www.lucintel.com/us-skincare-market-013-2018.aspx

CHAPTER 2
[1] Rippon I, Steptoe A. "Feeling Old vs Being Old, Associations Between Self-perceived Age and Mortality." JAMA Intern Med. 2015;175(2):307-309. doi: 10.1001/jamainternmed.2014.6580 https://jamanetwork.com/journals/jamainternalmedicine/fullarticle/2020288

[2] Ghodsbin F, Ahmadi ZS, Jahanbin I, Sharif F, "The Effects of Laughter Therapy on General Health of Elderly People Referring to Jahandidegan Community Center in Shiraz, Iran, 2014: A Randomized Controlled Trial." Int J Community Based Nurs Midwifery. 2015 Jan.; 3(1): 31–38. https://www.ncbi.nlm.nih.gov/pmc/articles/PMC4280555/

[3] Gagnon, et al. "Age-Specific Mortality During the 1918 Influenza Pandemic: Unravelling the Mystery of High Young Adult Mortality." PLoS One. 2013; 8(8): e69586. Aug. 5. 2013 doi: 10.1371/journal.pone.0069586. Online here.

[4] Okada HC, Alleyne B, Varghai K, Kinder K, Guyuron B. "Face It: Twins Who Smoke Look Older, Says Study in Plastic and Reconstructive Surgery." Plastic and Reconstructive Surgery (Nov. 2013; accessed Sept. 2017) 132(5):1085–1092 https://journals.lww.com/plasreconsurg/Abstract/2013/11000/Facial_Changes_Caused_by_Smoking___A_Comparison.10.aspx

[5] Chen Y, Lyga J. "Brain-Skin Connection: Stress, Inflammation and Skin Aging" (June 2014; accessed Sept. 2017) 13(3): 177–190. Inflammation and Allergy Drug Targets. Published doi: 10.2174/1871528113666140522104422

[6] Dhabhar FS, Ann NY. "Acute stress enhances while chronic stress suppresses skin immunity. The role of stress hormones and leukocyte trafficking." Acad Sci. (2000; accessed Oct. 2017) 917:876-93. https://www.ncbi.nlm.nih.gov/pubmed/11268419

[7] Lavretsky H, Newhouse PA. "Stress, Inflammation and Aging." American Journal of Geriatric Psychiatry. Sept. 2012; accessed Sept. 2017) 20(9): 729-733 doi: 10.1097/JGP.0b013e31826573cf

[8] Yokota M1, Tokudome Y. "The Effect of Glycation on Epidermal Lipid Content, Its Metabolism and Change in Barrier Function." Laboratory of Dermatological Physiology, Faculty of Pharmaceutical Sciences, Josai University, Sakado, Japan. Skin Pharmacol Physiol. (Epub Aug. 23, 2016; accessed Sept. 2017) 29(5):231-242. doi: 10.1159/000448121.

[9] Fowler SP, Williams K, Resendez RG, Hunt KJ, Hazuda HP, Stern MP. "Fueling the Obesity Epidemic? Artificially Sweetened Beverage Use and Long-term Weight Gain." Obesity A Research Journal (Sept. 06 2012; accessed Sept. 2017) 1894-1900 doi: https://doi.org/10.1038/oby.2008.284

[10] Lin JS, O'Connor E, Rossom RC, Perdue LA, Eckstrom E. "Screening for cognitive impairment in older adults: a systematic review for the U.S. Preventive Services Task Force." Ann Intern Med (2013; accessed Sept. 2017) 159:601-12

[11] Mayo Clinic Staff. "Alcohol: If You Drink, Keep It Moderate." Mayo Clinic. (Aug. 30 2016; accessed Oct. 2017) https://www.mayoclinic.org/healthy-lifestyle/nutrition-and-healthy-eating/in-depth/alcohol/art-20044551

[12] Clugston RD, Blaner WS. "The Adverse Effects Of Alcohol On Vitamin A Metabolism." Nutrients. (May 2012; accessed Oct. 2017) 4(5): 356–371. Epub 2012 May 7. doi: 10.3390/nu4050356

[13] Diaz-Gerevini GT, et al. "Beneficial action of resveratrol: How and why?" Nutrition. (Feb. 2016; accessed Oct. 2017) Epub Sept. 20, 2015 32:174. doi: 10.1016/j.nut.2015.08.017

[14] Center For Disease Control and Prevention. "Short Sleep Duration Among US Adults." (May 2, 2017; Oct. 2017) https://www.cdc.gov/sleep/data_statistics.html

[15] Oyetakin White P, Koo B, Matsui MS, Yarosh D, Fthenakis C, Cooper KD, Baron ED. "Effects of Sleep Quality on Skin Aging and Function." Department of Dermatology, Department of Pulmonary and Sleep Medicine, University Hospitals Case Medical Center and Case Western Reserve University, Cleveland, Ohio USA, and Estee Lauder Companies Inc., Melville, New York USA. (Sept. 30, 2014; accessed Oct. 2017) https://doi.org/10.1111/ced.12455

[16] Wolkowitz OM, Reus VI, Mellon SH. "Of Sound Mind And Body; Depression, Disease, and Accelerated Aging." Dialogues in Clinical Neuroscience. (Mar. 2011; accessed Nov. 2017) 13(1): 25–39 https://www.ncbi.nlm.nih.gov/pmc/articles/PMC3181963/

[17] Benros ME, Waltoft BL, Nordentoft M, et al. "Autoimmune Diseases and Severe Infections as Risk Factors for Mood Disorders A Nationwide Study." JAMA Psychiatry. (Aug. 2013; accessed Nov. 2017) 70(8):812-820. doi:10.1001/jamapsychiatry.2013.111

[18] Vegeto E, Benedusi V, Maggi A. "Estrogen anti-inflammatory activity in brain: a therapeutic opportunity for menopause and neurodegenerative diseases." Frontiers in Neuroendocrinology (Oct. 2008; accessed Nov. 2017) 29(4): 507-519

[19] Jameson LJ, et al. "Hypopituitarism and growth hormone deficiency." Endocrinology: Adult and Pediatric. 7th ed. Philadelphia, Pa.; Saunders Elsevier; (2016; accessed Oct. 2017) http://www.clinicalkey.com.

[20] Godfrey RJ, Madgwick Z, Whyte GP. "The exercise-induced growth hormone response in athletes." Sports Medicine. (2003; accessed Oct. 2017) 33(8):599-613. https://www.ncbi.nlm.nih.gov/pubmed/12797841

[21] Okada HC, Alleyne B, Varghai K, Kinder K, Guyuron B. "Facial Changes Caused By Smoking: A Comparison Between Smoking and Nonsmoking Identical Twins." Plastic Reconstructive Surgery. (Nov. 2013; accessed Nov. 2017) 132(5):1085-92. doi: 10.1097/PRS.0b013e3182a4c20a.

CHAPTER 3

[1] Sachdeva. "Fitzpatrick Skin typing: Applications in Dermatology." Indian Journal of Dermatology Venereol Leprol (Jan.-Feb. 2009; accessed Sept. 2017) 75(1):93-94 http://www.bioline.org.br/pdf?dv09029

[2] Lemperle G, Homes RE, Cohen SR, Lemperle SM. "A Classification of Facial Wrinkles." Plastic and Reconstructive Surgery. (Nov. 2001; accessed Dec. 2017) 108(6) https://www.researchgate.net/publication/11643185_A_Classification_of_Facial_Wrinkles

[3] Allergy Asthma Proc. 2017 July 1; 38(4): 294-299. doi: 10.2500/aap.2017.38.4055. Seasonal variation and monthly patterns of skin symptoms in Korean children with atopic eczema/dermatitis syndrome. Kim M, Kim YM, Lee JY, Yang HK, Kim H, Cho J, Ahn K, Kim J.; J Dermatol. 2001 May; 28(5): 244-7. Changes in the seasonal dependence of atopic dermatitis in Japan. Uenishi T1, Sugiura H, Uehara M. Department of Dermatology, Shiga University of Medical Science, Tsukinowa-cho, Seta, Otsu 520-2192, Japan.

CHAPTER 4
[1] Bleske-Rechek A, Lighthall M. "Attractiveness and Rivalry in Women's Friendships with Women" Human Nature (2010; accessed Dec. 2017) 21(1): 82

[2] Transparency Market Research. "Anti-aging Market (Anti-wrinkle products, Hair Color, Hair restoration treatment, Breast augmentation and Radio frequency devices) - Global Industry Analysis, Size, Share, Growth, Trends and Forecast, 2013 – 2019." (Jan. 2014; accessed Oct. 2017) https://www.transparencymarketresearch.com/anti-aging-market.html

[3] Boothroyd LG, Jucker J, Thornborrow T, Jamieson MA, Burt DM, Barton RA, Evans EH, Tovee MJ. "Television exposure predicts body size ideals in rural Nicaragua." British Journal of Psychology. (Feb. 22, 2016; accessed Dec. 2017) doi: 10.1111/bjop.12184

CHAPTER 6
[1] Nicas M, Best D. "A study quantifying the hand-to-face contact rate and its potential application to predicting respiratory tract infection." J Occup Environ Hyg. 2008 Jun.; 5(6):347-52. doi: 10.1080/15459620802003896.

[2] Ganceviciene R, Liakou AI, Theodoridis, A., Makrantonaki E, Zouboulis CC. "Skin anti-aging strategies" Dermatoendocrinol. 2012 Jul. 1; 4(3): 308–319. doi: 10.4161/derm.22804

[3] Addor, Flavia Alvim Sant'anna. Antioxidants in dermatology. Anais Brasileiros de Dermatologia, 2017 May-June; 92(3), 356-362. doi: 10.1590/abd1806-4841.20175697

[4] 52. Bissett DL, Miyamoto K, Sun P, Li J, Berge CA. Topical niacinamide reduces yellowing, wrinkling, red blotchiness, and hyperpigmented spots in aging facial skin. Int J Cosmet Sci. 2004; 26:231–8. doi: 10.1111/j.1467-2494.2004.00228.x. [PubMed] [Cross Ref]
53. Haftek M, Mac-Mary S, Le Bitoux MA, Creidi P, Seité S, Rougier A, et al. Clinical, biometric and structural evaluation of the long-term effects of a topical treatment with ascorbic acid and madecassoside in photoaged human skin. Exp Dermatol. 2008; 17:946–52. doi: 10.1111/j.1600-0625.2008.00732.x. [PubMed] [Cross Ref]

[5] Draelos ZD, Ertel K, Berge C. "Niacinamide-containing facial moisturizer improves skin barrier and benefits subjects with rosacea." Cutis. 2005 Aug;76(2):135-41.

[6] Draelos ZD, Ertel K, Berge C. "Niacinamide-containing facial moisturizer improves skin barrier and benefits subjects with rosacea." Cutis. 2005 Aug;76(2):135-41.

[7] Navindra P. Seeram, Michael Aviram, Yanjun Zhang, Susanne M. Henning, Lydia Feng, Mark Dreher and David Heber. "Comparison of Antioxidant Potency of Commonly Consumed Polyphenol-Rich Beverages in the United States" Center for Human Nutrition, David Geffen School of Medicine, University of California, Los

Angeles, California 90095; Lipid Research Laboratory, Technion Faculty of Medicine, Rambam Medical Center, Haifa, Israel; and POM Wonderful, LLC, Los Angeles, California 90064 J. Agric. Food Chem., 2008, 56 (4), pp 1415–1422 doi: 10.1021/ jf073035s

[8] Palombo P, Fabrizi G, Ruocco V, Ruocco E, Fluhr J, Roberts R, Morganti P. "Beneficial Long-Term Effects of Combined Oral/Topical Antioxidant Treatment with the Carotenoids Lutein and Zeaxanthin on Human Skin: A Double-Blind, Placebo-Controlled Study." Skin Pharmacol Physiol 2007;20:199-210. doi: 10.1159/000101807 https://content.karger.com/Article/Abstract/101807

[9] Zussman J, Ahdout J, Kim J. "Vitamins and photoaging: Do scientific data support their use?" J Am Acad Dermatol. 2010 Sep;63(3):507-25. doi: 10.1016/j. jaad.2009.07.037.

[10] Nair R, Maseeh A. "Vitamin D: The "sunshine" vitamin." J Pharmacol Pharmacother. 2012;3(2):118-26. https://www.ncbi.nlm.nih.gov/pmc/articles/ PMC3356951/

[11] Lim HW, Arellano-Mendoza MI, Stengel F, "Detroit, Michigan; Mexico City, Mexico: Buenos Aires, Argentina: Current Challenges in photoprotection"

[12] Wang SQ, Dusza SW, Lim HW. "New York, New York and Detroit Michigan: Safety of retinyl palmitate in sunscreens: a critical analysis"

[13] https://www.health.harvard.edu/diseases-and-conditions/benefits-of-moderate-sun-exposure

[14] Christensen D. "Data Still Cloudy on Association Between Sunscreen Use and Melanoma Risk" JNCI: Journal of the National Cancer Institute, Volume 95, Issue 13, 2 July 2003, Pages 932–933, https://doi.org/10.1093/jnci/95.13.932

[15] Schneider D, Dennerlein K, Göen T, Schaller KH, Drexler H, Korinth G. "Influence of artificial sebum on the dermal absorption of chemicals in excised human skin: A proof-of-concept study." Toxicol In Vitro. 2016 Jun;33:23-8. doi: 10.1016/j.tiv.2016.02.010.

[16] Draelos, Z.D. "Cosmetic Dermatology: Products and Procedures, Second Edition" Wiley-Blackwell, Dec. 2015

[17] Peng Y, Glattauer V, Werkmeister JA, Ramshaw JAM. "Evaluation for collagen products for cosmetic application."

[18] https://www.aad.org/practicecenter/quality/clinical-guidelines/atopic-dermatitis/ topical-therapy

[19] Eichenfeld, et al. "Guidelines for the care and management of atopic dermatitis." JAAD July 2014, 71:1.

[20] Meckfessel MH, Brandt S. "The structure, function, and importance of ceramides in skin and their use as therapeutic agents in skin-care products." J Am Acad Dermatol. 2014 Jul;71(1):177-84. doi: 10.1016/j.jaad.2014.01.891.

[21] Draelos ZD, DiNardo JC. "A re-evaluation of the comedogenicity concept." J Am Acad Dermatol. 2006 Mar;54(3):507-12.; Morris W.E. and Kwan S.C. "Use of the Rabbit Ear Model in Evaluating Comedogenic Potential in Cosmetic Ingredients", Revlon Research Center, Received Oct. 1981 J. Soc. Cosmet. Chem., 34, 215-225 (Aug. 1983)

[22] Mukherjee S, Date A, Patravale V, et al. "Retinoids in cosmeceuticals." Dermatol Ther 2006; 19; 289-96

[23] Noy N. Interactions of retinoids with lipid bilayers and with membranes. In: Liverea M. Packer L eds. Retinoids. New York: Marcel Dekker 1993; 17-27; Bailly J, Crettaz M, Schifflers MH, et al. "In vitro metabolism by human skin and fibroblasts of retinol, retinal and retinoic acid." Exp Dermatol 1998; 7(1): 27-34.; Darlenski R, Surber C, Fluhr JW. "Topical retinoids in the management of photodamaged skin: from theory to evidence-based practical approach" Br J Dermatol 2010; 163:1157-65; Sorg O, Antille C, Kaya G, et al. "Retinoids in cosmeceuticals." Dermatol Therapy 2006; 19; 289-296)

[24] McCook JP. "Topical Products for the Aging Face." Clin Plastic Surg 43 (2016) 597-604

[25] Smit JV, de Jong EM, de Jongh GJ, van de Kerkhof PC. "Topical all-trans retinoic acid does not influence minimal erythema doses for UVB light in normal skin." Acta Derm Venereol. 2000 Jan-Feb;80(1):66-7.

[26] Keyes BE, Liu S, Asare A, et al. "Impaired Epidermal to Dendritic T Cell Signaling Slows Wound Repair in Aged Skin." Cell, 2016; 167 (5): 1323 doi: 10.1016/j. cell.2016.10.052; Brice E. Keyes, Siqi Liu, Amma Asare, Shruti Naik, John Levorse, Lisa Polak, Catherine P. Lu, Maria Nikolova, Hilda Amalia Pasolli, Elaine Fuchs. Impaired Epidermal to Dendritic T Cell Signaling Slows Wound Repair in Aged Skin. Cell, 2016; 167 (5): 1323 DOI: 10.1016/j.cell.2016.10.052

[27] Lodish H, Berk A, Zipursky SL, et al. "Collagen: The Fibrous Proteins of the Matrix." Molecular Cell Biology. 4th edition. New York: W. H. Freeman; 2000. Section 22.3, https://www.ncbi.nlm.nih.gov/books/NBK21582/

[28] Fitzpatrick, Richard & Rostan, Elizabeth. (2003). "Reversal of photodamage with topical growth factors: A pilot study." Journal of cosmetic and laser therapy:

official publication of the European Society for Laser Dermatology. 5. 25-34. 10.1080/14764170305499; Gold MH, Goldman MP, Biron J. "Efficacy of novel skin cream containing mixture of human growth factors and cytokines for skin rejuvenation." J Drugs Dermatol. 2007 Feb;6(2):197-201.; Mehta, Rahul & Fitzpatrick, Richard. (2006). "Endogenous growth factors as cosmeceuticals". Dermatologic therapy. 2007 Sep-Oct;20(5):350-9.; Gold, Michael & Goldman, Mitchel & Biron, Julie. (2007). "Human growth factor and cytokine skin cream for facial skin rejuvenation as assessed by 3D in vivo optical skin imaging". Journal of drugs in dermatology: 2007 Oct;6(10):1018-23.; Mehta, Rahul & Smith, Stacy & Grove, Gary & O Ford, Rosanne & Canfield, William & Donofrio, Lisa & C Flynn, Timothy & J Leyden, James. (2008). "Reduction in facial photodamage by a topical growth factor product". Journal of drugs in dermatology, 2008 Sep;7(9):864-71.; Sundaram, Hema & Mehta, Rahul & A Norine, Josie & Kircik, Leon & E Cook-Bolden, Fran & H Atkin, Deborah & Werschler, Wm & Fitzpatrick, Richard. (2009). "Topically Applied Physiologically Balanced Growth Factors: A New Paradigm of Skin Rejuvenation". Journal of drugs in dermatology: 2009 May;8(5 Suppl Skin Rejuvenation):4-13.

[29] Newman, H "Ethanol signals for apoptosis in cultured skin cells." Apr. 2002.

[30] Erdman SE, Poutahidis T. "Probiotic 'glow of health': it's more than skin deep." Benef Microbes. 2014;5(2):109-19. https://www.ncbi.nlm.nih.gov/pmc/articles/PMC4354898/

[31] Farris PK. "Are skincare products with probiotics worth the hype?" http://www.dermatologytimes.com/dermatology/are-skincare-products-probiotics-worth-hype

CHAPTER 7
[1] Pesce NL. "Kim Kardashian's $1,500 'vampire facial' is a Hollywood hit that promises younger, firmer-looking skin" https://www.nydailynews.com/life-style/health/kim-kardashian-vampire-facelift-bloody-mess-article-1.1285646

[2] Li WH, Fassih A, Binner C, Parsa R, Southall MD. "Low-level red LED light inhibits hyperkeratinization and inflammation induced by unsaturated fatty acid in an in vitro model mimicking acne." Lasers Surg Med. (Feb. 2018; accessed Jan. 2018) 50(2):158-165. doi: 10.1002/lsm.22747.

CHAPTER 8
[1] Acne.org. "Light Therapy – Blue and/or Red Light Therapy." (Feb. 23, 2018; accessed Mar. 2018) https://www.acne.org/light-therapy.html

CHAPTER 11
[1] "2016 Cosmetic Plastic Surgery Statistics" American Society of Plastic Surgeons https://www.plasticsurgery.org/documents/News/Statistics/2016/cosmetic-procedure-

trends-2016.pdf

[2] "2016 Cosmetic Plastic Surgery Statistics" American Society of Plastic Surgeons
https://www.plasticsurgery.org/documents/News/Statistics/2016/2016-plastic-surgery-statistics-report.pdf

[3] "2016 Cosmetic Plastic Surgery Statistics" American Society of Plastic Surgeons
https://www.plasticsurgery.org/news/press-releases/new-statistics-reveal-the-shape-of-plastic-surgery

CHAPTER 12
[1] Ozog DM, Moy RL. "A Randomized Split-Scar Study of Intraoperative Treatment of Surgical Wound Edges to Minimize Scarring." Arch Dermatol. 2011;147(9):1108–1110. doi:10.1001/archdermatol.2011.248

CHAPTER 13
[1] "New Statistics Reflecting the Changing Face of Plastic Surgery" American Society of Plastic Surgeons. Feb 25, 2016 [Press Release]
https://www.plasticsurgery.org/news/press-releases/new-statistics-reflect-the-changing-face-of-plastic-surgery

DR. JENNIFER JANIGA

Made in the USA
Columbia, SC
03 November 2020